ANNUAL REVIEW of
Nursing Research

Volume 1, 1983

ANNUAL REVIEW of Nursing Research

Volume 1, 1983

Harriet H. Werley, Ph.D.
Joyce J. Fitzpatrick, Ph.D.
Editors

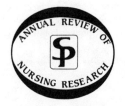

SPRINGER PUBLISHING COMPANY
New York

Springer Publishing Company, Inc.
200 Park Avenue South
New York, New York 10003

84 85 86 87 88 / 10 9 8 7 6 5 4 3 2 1
ISBN 0-8261-4350-4
ISSN 0739–6686

Printed in the United States of America

Contents

Preface

In the process of maturing, most disciplines develop media to review critically, on a regular basis, the work that leads the discipline forward, so that students, faculty, and other scholars can recognize the advances made, the existing gaps, and the areas that need further work. Nursing had not followed this tradition until recently, when reviews of literature in a particular problem area began appearing in journals such as *Nursing Research* and *Research in Nursing and Health*. Useful as they are for broad overviews on selected topics, these articles, however, do not generally follow the pattern of *critical,* integrative reviews designed to help scholars identify what has been done, what has been done well, what has not been done well, what are the gaps, and what are the suggested directions for the field. The function of systematic, critical assessment of advances in a field is usually assumed by a regular Annual Review. Such a medium has been lacking in the discipline of nursing. With the present volume, nursing obtains its own medium of scholarly advances, the *Annual Review of Nursing Research*.

In some disciplines, annual reviews encompass problems, issues, advances, and research. For a field such as nursing, an annual review as comprehensive as that could become so large and overwhelming that it might simply be another volume resting on a reference shelf. For nursing, in the judgement of the senior editor of this newly created medium, a review should be limited to research pertinent to nursing and health, and should result in a systematic assessment of knowledge development. Thus, it would also be more likely to provide nursing with an appropriate data-based foundation.

The genesis of this comprehensive publishing project extended over a dozen years. In the late 1960s and early 1970s, Harriet Werley began discussing the plan with colleagues and friends, eliciting their reactions to the idea of creating an *Annual Review of Nursing Research,* and also seeking suggestions about how the volumes might be organized—either by the traditional clinical content areas, by concepts being taught, or by some other format. Werley continued to discuss the plan with many individuals in private and at conferences, as well as at meetings of the Executive Committee of the American Nurses' Association (ANA) Council of Nurse Researchers (CNR) during the years 1976 to 1980. She presented a motion to the membership of the CNR at one of their business meetings to see if there would be support for the idea of developing a series of reviews. The vote was in the affirmative and she was encouraged to proceed. At several annual meetings she reported back to this body on the progress being made, which was usually very slow, apparently because nursing really was not ready for this move; the amount of research for review in any one area of nursing was not yet voluminous.

In the early 1980s, Werley began to sense that she was getting a different reaction. Many nurses recognized the value of the suggested project and were eager to contribute their thoughts. In 1979, prior to leaving the position as Associate Dean for Research at the University of Illinois College of Nursing, she decided to assemble faculty colleagues from the different nursing areas so she might profit from their ideas and reactions. These colleagues were tremendously interested and did not want to drop the subject without more discussion; thus, a second session was held.

Joyce Fitzpatrick accepted Werley's invitation to become coeditor and shared with her the conceptual foundations and much of the practical work that preceded this complex project. Roma Lee Taunton, a research extern and a doctoral student from the University of Kansas Educational Psychology and Research Program, was engaged to scrutinize the notes and materials collected for discussion at the first working session of the editors in March 1981. This led to the formulation of the first five-year plan for the proposed annual review, suggestions of persons to be invited for the Advisory Board, and eventually the identificaton of authors for the first three volumes. Dr. Ursula Springer, President of Springer Publishing Company, was a source of encouragement, and she expressed interest in publishing the *Annual Review of Nursing Research*. The editors conducted much of their business with colleagues at various regional and national meetings, as well as by phone, and by September 1981 all authors for Volume 1 were commissioned for their chapters.

In developing the master plan, the editors were guided by the many reactions and suggestions elicited from fellow nurses. It was decided that each volume would contain at least four parts: Research on Nursing Practice, Research on Nursing Care Delivery, Research on Nursing Education, and Research on the Profession of Nursing. The parts would be composed of chapters, with about five chapters included under Nursing Practice. The chapters under Nursing Practice for Volume 1 would pertain to human development throughout the life span; for Volume 2,* the emphasis of these

*Readers can get a preview of the planned chapters for Volume 2 from the Table of Contents included in this volume.

chapters would be on the family; and for Volume 3, on the community. The research reviewed in these volumes would be useful to practitioners, administrators, and educators. The volumes, therefore, would be appealing to all groups of nurses, as well as to others interested in nursing and health.

For some volumes there may be an additional part with chapters presented as stimulus pieces. If the research in a particular area is sparse but very much needed, an author may review critically the existing studies and then put the emphasis on future directions and stimulating research in that area. Also, a foreign research colleague may be invited to review the nursing research in her/his country for the benefit of international perspectives in nursing research.

In this first volume, as can be noted from the Table of Contents, the research reviewed pertains to five areas of human development along the life span from infants to the elderly and dying persons. Kathryn E. Barnard reviewed nursing research related to infants and young children; Mary J. Denyes dealt with schoolage children; Joanne Sabol Stevenson's content was the adult; Mary Opal Wolanin was concerned with clinical nursing research pertaining to the elderly; and, Jeanne Quint Benoliel dealt with death, dying, and terminal illness. In the area of research on nursing care delivery both the intra- and interorganizational aspects were covered. Ada Sue Hinshaw and Jan R. Atwood addressed aspects of nursing staff turnover, stress, and satisfaction, while Janelle C. Krueger reviewed research pertaining to nursing interorganizational relations. In the area of research on the profession of nursing, Mary E. Conway reviewed studies relating to socialization into the profession and some aspects of roles in nursing. A stimulus piece, the chapter on philosophic inquiry developed by Rosemary Ellis, represents an important yet underdeveloped area that we hope will grow. Unfortunately, as often happens with the first volume of an annual, some of the commissioned chapters were not completed. These gaps in presentation will be remedied in future volumes.

No venture like that of establishing an annual review can be accomplished without the contributions of many, many individuals, ranging from those nurses who initially listened and offered suggestions, to Dr. Ursula Springer, President of Springer Publishing Company, who provided consistent support and practical advice. Much credit goes to the Advisory Board members, who assisted with the review of manuscripts; the authors, a number of whom are Advisory Board members, who were brave enough to take on the new kind of writing—a critical, integrative review of research; the secretaries—who assisted the senior editor in keeping the simultaneous work on three volumes straight—Theresa Terry, later Juanita Black at the University of Missouri-Columbia School of Nursing, and more recently Catherine R. Sweet at the University of Wisconsin-Milwaukee School of Nursing; and those who provided assistance for the coeditor at the Case Western Reserve University School of Nursing—Sara Pencil, Loretta Crenshaw, and most of all, Bertha Willis.

Reader reactions to the volumes as they appear will be appreciated; suggestions are desired, as are expressions of interest in contributing a chapter in an area of one's expertise. Authors are selected mainly from those conducting research; they are recognized, creditable investigators, qualified to evaluate the research in an area. Suggestions from both the Advisory Board and authors are especially welcome because their comments stem from involvement and first-hand knowledge of the operations.

Contributors

Jan R. Atwood, Ph.D.
College of Nursing
University of Arizona
Tucson, Arizona

Kathryn E. Barnard, Ph.D.
School of Nursing
University of Washington
Seattle, Washington

Jeanne Quint Benoliel, D.N.Sc.
School of Nursing
University of Washington
Seattle, Washington

Mary E. Conway, Ph.D.
School of Nursing
Medical College of Georgia
Augusta, Georgia

Mary J. Denyes, Ph.D.
College of Nursing
Wayne State University
Detroit, Michigan

Rosemary Ellis, Ph.D.
School of Nursing
Case Western Reserve University
Cleveland, Ohio

Ada Sue Hinshaw, Ph.D.
College of Nursing
University of Arizona
Tucson, Arizona

Janelle C. Krueger, Ph.D.
School of Nursing
University of Colorado
Denver, Colorado

Joanne Sabol Stevenson, Ph.D.
School of Nursing
The Ohio State University
Columbus, Ohio

Mary Opal Wolanin, M.P.A.
College of Nursing
University of Arizona
Tucson, Arizona

Forthcoming

ANNUAL REVIEW OF
NURSING RESEARCH, Volume 2

Tentative Contents

PART I

Research on Nursing Practice

CHAPTER 1

Nursing Research Related to Infants and Young Children

KATHRYN E. BARNARD

SCHOOL OF NURSING

UNIVERSITY OF WASHINGTON

CONTENTS

SELECTED HEALTH PROBLEMS

There is a timeliness to the publication of an annual review in nursing. This review was focused on nursing research about children under 5 years of age. The review included the nursing identified publications reviewed by Medlars for the five-year period, 1977 to 1981; it was not possible to retrieve all nursing-authored studies in publications if they were not identified as

Acknowledgment is given to Rebecca Kang, Georgina Sumner, Etsuko Kimura, Marian Cole, and Verna Smith, whose assistance in preparing this chapter contributed at each phase of the process.

3

nursing. The review was challenging for several reasons. With the exception of *Nursing Research, Research in Nursing and Health,* and the *Maternal Child Nursing Journal,* most nursing publications do not have a standard research reporting style. In addition, there are studies about isolated topics or issues that are hard to fit into a thematic whole.

The American Nurses' Association's (1981) definition of nursing as the diagnosis and treatment of human responses to health problems was used as a framework for reviewing the nursing literature. The health problems selected were prematurity, attachment, hospitalization, and growth-fostering environments. The studies cited in this review were judged to make a substantial contribution to the literature because of the questions the investigators asked about responses of infants and children to the four targeted health problems. There is no claim that all the studies are methodologically sound; in fact, few of the studies approach the criterion of providing generalizable results.

The literature portrays a developing science seeking answers to numerous questions about children and their families. The major effort of this review was directed at describing the themes of the research and addressing whether the right questions were being asked; minimal attention was given to the issues of design and analysis. The studies reported in this chapter, while both of descriptive and experimental design, tend to have small samples and need to be replicated or expanded.

PREMATURITY

Over the past decade, advances in the science of neonatology have made it possible to improve the survival rate of premature infants. Immaturity of body systems prevents optimal responses from preterm infants to an independent extrauterine existence. A review of literature for the past five years indicated that nurses have been concerned with questions about how premature infants respond to extrauterine living and how nursing action influences the response and well-being of premature infants.

Infant Responses to Extrauterine Living

A promising area of research devoted to the question of the premature infant's response to respiratory therapy was the work by Collins (1978), who demonstrated that survival was enhanced by decreases in heart rate at least three hours after respiratory therapy was initiated. These results indicated that therapy was successful as tissues were perfused with oxygen, causing the heart rate to decrease. Another study using heart rate as an indicator was an investigation reported by Neal (1979). Infants between 31 and 36 weeks of gestation were exposed to an 80-decibel, low-intensity, auditory stimulus for 20 seconds, for a total of 30 trials. Heart rate response was sampled at successive 2-second intervals, before and after onset of the stimulus. Infants at 31 weeks of gestation showed heart rate deceleration to the stimulus, while 32- to 36-week-gestation infants demonstrated comparable patterns of acceleration followed by deceleration. The Neal work, while considered a pilot study, was cited because, along with the work of Collins (1978), it serves as a reminder that basic physiological measures such as heart rate can serve as important response indicators for the immature infant. In the first instance, Collins used heart rate as an indicator of the efficiency of the cardiorespiratory system. The mean hourly rate was used, taken retrospectively from clinical records. In the second study reported by Neal (1979), heart rate was measured in a more precise way; it was used to determine if immature infants have an orienting response to a novel stimulus. The heart rate was monitored before and after the stimulus presentation. While it may not be possible to measure orientation by the heart rate response in preterm infants, since there is little vagal control of the heart, the differential response patterns Neal described would be important for further investigation.

Nursing Actions to Influence the Response

In a series of studies, a group of investigators focused on infant sucking as a measure of the self-regulatory response. Descriptive studies showed that suction pressure while sucking was correlated positively with birth weight, gestational age, and health status (Ellison, Vidyasagar, & Anderson, 1979). Proposing that sucking stimulates physiological function, Anderson and Vidyasagar (1979) gave premature infants, $31.2 \pm .9$ weeks of gestation, finger sucking opportunities twice a day with 6- to 12-hour intervals between measures of the sucking response. Clinical sucking scores in this study were not correlated with birth weight or gestational age, but were correlated positively with blood pH and negatively with pCO_2 and serum bilirubin levels. These finger-sucking experiences seemed, from the investigators' observations, to promote neuromuscular coordination, alert activity, alert inactivity, and deep sleep.

    In another study, Measal and Anderson (1979) reported that sucking during and after tube feedings advanced the readiness for bottle feeding by 3 to 4 days; these infants gained 2.6 grams more per day and were discharged from the hospital 4 days earlier than infants who did not experience the sucking protocol. Anderson, Dahm, Ellis, and Vidyasagar (Note 1) next reported that a sequence of sucking opportunities before tube feedings did not influence the sucking pressure or the amount of arousal of preterm infants, as they had predicted. The investigators speculated whether these findings may have resulted from offering sucking experiences at times not contingent with the state of consciousness of the infants. This series of studies on the sucking response demonstrates the critical value of capitalizing on innate responses of preterm infants to facilitate their well-being. The question being investigated about sucking as a regulator of the infant's physiological and behavioral responses is a highly significant one for nursing and medical care of premature infants.

The question of how behavior of infants born prematurely is regulated by the external environment has been addressed by other investigators. It was hypothesized that early exposure to a neonatal environment characterized by predominantly noxious, varied, excessive, and unpredictable stimuli was a cause of abnormal behavior (Barnard, 1972). The striking absence of intrauterine-like stimulation, such as maternal heartbeat sounds and kinesthetic stimuli from maternal movement, prompted scientists to test the effects of tactile, auditory, kinesthetic, and/or visual stimulation on preterm infants.

Investigators tested the effects of single stimulus modalities as well as combinations of stimuli on the preterm infant. Kramer, Chamorro, Green, and Knudtson (1975) found that gentle, nonrhythmic stroking of the infant's body surface daily while the infant was hospitalized improved the rate of social development while there was no difference in cortisal levels, physical, motor, or mental development. Rice (1979) instructed mothers of infants who had been born prematurely to give their babies systematic stroking and massaging during the first four months after hospital discharge. The stimulated infants made significant gains in neurological development, weight gain, and mental development in comparison to those infants who did not receive the stimulation protocol.

Auditory stimulation was tested as a method for enhancing the quality of the Isolette environment. Chapman (1978, 1979) studied the effect of maternal voice recordings with a Brahms lullaby on the gross limb activity of experimental premature infants between 26 and 32 weeks of gestation. She hypothesized that patterned auditory stimulation would promote central nervous system maturation, which would in turn inhibit motor discharge. No significant differences were found between the experimental and control groups; however, data results were in the hypothesized direction. Malloy (1979) investigated the clinical effects of the same subjects exposed to maternal voice recordings and Brahms lullaby. Stimulated infants demonstrated faster weight gain in the hospital than control infants. The program did not have lasting effects; motor and mental developmental testing at 9 months of age demonstrated no difference between groups.

Other nurse scientists have combined two or more modalities of stimulation to influence the course of social, motor, and mental development. Rausch (1981) applied massage and passive range of motion exercises to preterm infants who weighed 1,000 to 2,000 grams at birth. Stimulated infants received this program once a day for 15 minutes during the first 10 days after birth. The infants in the experimental group had more stools on days 5 to 10, more caloric intake on days 6 to 10, and more daily weight gain than infants who were unstimulated. Barnard and Bee (Note 2) reported the results of manipulating the timing and contingency of a rocking-heartbeat stimulation program on the physical, neurological, and mental development of premature infants recruited into the study at less than 34 weeks of gestation. The variation of the timing and contingency of the stimulation was as follows: fixed interval, rocking-heartbeat stimulation for 15 minutes every hour; self-activated, the same rocking-heartbeat stimulation, triggered by the infant's own activity level; quasi-self-activated, infant-triggered stimulation but only when stimulation had not occurred in the previous 45 minutes. A control group received the normal hospital care. Results indicated that stimulation for all timing and contingency conditions reduced activity during the treatment period significantly more for the self-activated group than for the other treatment groups. Long term results demonstrated higher mental development for treatment versus control subjects at 24 months, with the quasi-self-activated group showing significantly higher mental scores than the fixed interval or self-activated subjects (Barnard & Bee, Note 3).

Investigations of the influences of external stimulation on behavior and well-being of the preterm infant provided no conclusive evidence. The studies of auditory stimulation, in which infant activity was used as a dependent measure (Chapman, 1978, 1979; Barnard & Bee, Note 2) demonstrated the same trend, stimulation reduced motor activity. Barnard and Bee (Note 2) also used motion stimulation. Greater weight gain was cited as a result of stimulation by Malloy (1979), Rice (1979), and Rausch (1981), but not by Kramer et al. (1975) or Barnard and Bee (Note 2). The investigation showing the most generalized change based on a stimulation program was reported by Rice (1979). There were gains for the experimental group in physical growth, neurological performance, and mental development. It is instructive to note two differences in the study by Rice. First, the stimulation occurred after the infants were discharged from the hospital, and second, the stimulation, stroking and massaging, was done by the mother. While there have been no published implications of the Rice work, it is still instructive to postulate that external stimulation might be more effective after the infant has stabilized physiologically, or if the stimulation specifically helps the infant regulate physiological function. It is in the latter case that the work of Anderson and Vidyasagar (1979) on sucking as a means of self-regulation is important.

With regard to the second difference in the stimulation used by Rice, the mother gave the program; this feature resulted in a treatment that was much more complex since it involved all the specifics of both the massaging and the dynamics of dyadic instruction. The results Barnard and Bee (Note 2) cited are related; the best long term mental development was for premature infants who had the rocking and heartbeat stimulation contingent on both their activity and a discrimination task of learning when they could and could not activate the stimulation. Therefore, while the past research has not given clear answers about whether external stimuli influence the response of preterm infants, investigators can now begin to ask more specific questions. Three important ones to address are: How do external stimuli influence self-regulation? How do the complexity and responsiveness of the stimuli influence the infants' responses? How do external stimuli influence stabilized versus unstabilized infants?

Research is needed to identify reliable and valid infant reponses. Besides the responses of sucking, neurological reflexes, and heart rate, longitudinal investigation is needed to trace the evolution of crying, motor movement, seeing, hearing, and state organization. Descriptive studies are needed to identify nursing actions focused on cardiovascular care, pulmonary care, maintenance of skin integrity, promotion of optimal nutrition, sensory and motor development, bowel and bladder maintenance, temperature regulation, and promotion of rest and comfort, as well as management of pain of premature infants.

Finally, a series of nursing studies is needed to evaluate the effect of nursing action on preterm infant well-being. Possible areas of research are the influence on infant activity of the caregiving in the neonatal intensive care environment, consolidation of procedures to facilitate uninterrupted periods of rest, timing of stimulation programs according to emerging infant responses, comparative effects of hospital-based stimulation programs and home-based programs, and the properties influencing the transaction between parent and infant.

ATTACHMENT

Parents develop a sense of wanting to protect the young child from harm. The importance of love and care to the young child was demonstrated by Spitz (1950), Bowlby (1969), and Casler (1961).

There are two issues concerning attachment: how the young child develops a sense of trust and safety in the caregiver, and how the parent develops a sense of needing to protect the young. Bowlby (1969) clearly stated the biological significance of the attachment relationship—there is a protector and a protectee; the young, the sick, and the dependent need to have an attachment relationship to survive.

Parent to Child

Nursing research from 1977 to 1981 dealt almost exclusively with the question of parent to child attachment. Reva Rubin (1977) discussed this process in relation to "binding-in." She identified the binding-in process as active, intermittent, and accumulative, occurring over the last trimester of pregnancy and for the first 12 to 15 months following birth. Rubin differentiated the stages of this process. First the mother is aware of "Another." "There is a psychosocial as well as biological interdependent reciprocity, or symbiosis, between mother and child during pregnancy (p. 67). After delivery the binding-in changed form. Postdelivery "there is an identification of the infant as a human entity with its own form, appearance, and behavior" (p. 68). During the postpartum period, a polarization of selves begins. Rubin described competing forces, with the force to be one contrasted to the force to separate. This complexity is central to the resolution of the parent's attachment to the infant. The nursing studies reviewed addressed all of the processes proposed by Rubin: the symbiosis, identification, polarization, and particularly the identification of the infant as a separate person; however, few nurse investigators cited Rubin's formulation as a basis for their work. Recognition of the conceptual and theoretical origins of research questions must be a more conscious behavior of investigators.

Curry (1982) addressed the question of mother-infant closeness as it related to promoting reciprocity; she followed the leads of previous work by Klaus, Jerauld, Kreger, McAlpine, Steffa, and Kennell (1972) and De Chateau (1976). Curry promoted extended skin-to-skin contact for 15 minutes following delivery for the experimental group; there were no differences in attachment behaviors when measured 36 hours after delivery and at 3 months of age. Curry's sample consisted of married, financially stable, well-educated mothers, who were well prepared for the childbirth experience. Possibly these mothers had already achieved the interdependent reciprocity during their pregnancy, and this stage of binding-in had been achieved. Curry's findings raise questions about other studies, where investigators found increased expression of maternal attachment with close extended contact immediately following delivery (De Chateau, 1976; Klaus et al., 1972; Klaus & Kennell, 1970). Perhaps the issue of immediate contact is important for mothers who have not developed this interdependent reciprocity during pregnancy. A prenatal attachment scale published by Cranley (1981) will make it possible to identify mothers who have achieved reciprocity during pregnancy. Once the identification is made, the effect of extended contact can be tested, considering the differences in the mothers at the time of delivery with respect to reciprocity.

A study by Carter-Jessop (1981) is noteworthy. This investigator conducted an experiment attempting both to influence the reciprocity of the mother and fetus and to promote identification of the fetal parts. During the last trimester mothers were instructed at their prenatal medical checkups to identify the fetal head, legs, and back by tactile exploration of their abdomen. The mothers were encouraged to identify how their actions influenced the fetus: how the infant responded when the mother was more active, went to sleep, and when the mother touched a fetal part. In observations made postpartum about the mothers' behavior toward their infants, Carter-Jessop found that mothers in the experimental group did more proximity-seeking and had more interaction with the infants than mothers who did not have this guidance and experience. This small-sample study needs replication. The procedure and timing during the last trimester of pregnancy dealt precisely with what Rubin (1977) identified as the binding-in task during pregnancy—being able to comprehend the interdependent reciprocity. The prenatal nursing action such as proposed by Carter-Jessop's work would be an important therapy to test and to contrast with a protocol such as Curry's (1982) of promoting maternal-infant contact postpartum.

A number of nurse investigators have tried to influence the parent's awareness of the infant's individuality. This is precisely the task that Rubin (1977) identified as prominent in the period after delivery and extending through the first weeks. In studies done at the University of Washington, Ryan (1973) and Kang (1974) used the Brazelton Neonatal Assessment Scale (Brazelton, 1973). This scale, which examines a newborn's behavioral responsiveness, was used as the basis for sharing with parents that babies, and in particular their baby, could see, hear, respond, and be consoled when upset. The samples for both studies were small, but the results encouraged subsequent investigators to pursue further experiments. Their findings indicated that parents who had the information about their own infant's behavior responded more positively about their infant and used a greater range of comforting strategies for infant distress at 1 month.

Anderson (1981) reported a study that extended this strategy. Thirty middle-class, primiparous mothers of female infants were assigned randomly to three treatment comparison groups. Two of the groups received information about their infant. One group had the investigator tell them about their infant's behavior following the investigator's examination of the infant with the Neonatal Behavioral Assessment Scale. The second group of mothers had the chance to observe the investigator examine their infant on the items of the Neonatal Behavioral Assessment Scale. The third group received information about purchasing and using various infant products; they did not have any information about their infant's behavior. The Price Adaptation Scale (Note 4) was used to observe maternal infant reciprocity at 10 days of age. Reciprocity as defined in the scale was a relationship consisting of mutuality, adaptation, sensitivity, enjoyment, and pleasure. There were differences between the groups. The mothers who had their infant's behaviors demonstrated to them had higher scores on the maternal reciprocity cluster, and infants in both the infant behavior information and the demonstration groups showed higher scores on the infant cluster. There were no differences on the interaction cluster, thus suggesting that while the mother and infant were independently more active in the transaction, there was no difference in the amount of interaction.

Father-Infant Relationship

In at least two studies, investigators tested methods of influencing the father-infant relationship. Pannabecker and Emde (1977) tested instruction to new fathers about physical characteristics of infants and infant exercise and gave the fathers an opportunity for interaction with their infants during the first day and a half. Other fathers had an additional session where the investigator demonstrated their infants' behavioral responsiveness. Fathers in the control group received no instruction or time with infant for demonstration. At 4 weeks the fathers were observed interacting with their infants during a physical examination. There were no differences in the fathers' behavior with the infants at that observation. All fathers were white, middle-class, and pregnancy was considered normal.

Jones (1981) investigated how fathers and infants get to know each other. Thirty-four of 51 fathers held their infants in the first hour; 17 did not. The decision was the father's and not influenced in any way by the design of the study. Follow-up at 1 month postpartum revealed that fathers who had initially held their baby demonstrated more nonverbal behavior toward their infant. Nonverbal behaviors included eye-to-eye contact, smile, active touch, kiss/nuzzle, hold/move/support, and vigorous kinesthetic stimulation.

In reviewing these investigations about parental attachment, the question of dependent measures must be addressed. What is a valid measure of parental attachment or binding-in? Is it seeking of physical proximity? Is it responding to the distress of the infant? Is it providing care for the dependent individual? Is it reciprocal interactions? Is it having a positive view of the infant? Is it having a positive view of self? Is it satisfaction with the caregiving role? If we were to depend on Bowlby's (1969) concepts, it would be the parent's protection of the baby and response to distress. Ainsworth (1973) would compel us to look also at proximity-seeking. Rubin (1977) would direct us to measure the identification of the infant as an individual and the parent's self-identity, as well as the reciprocal interdependence. In further investigations it would be important to be more specific about the theoretical basis for the design and measures.

An interesting study was presented by Holaday (1981, 1982). She studied crying behaviors of chronically ill infants and their mothers' responses to the crying. She found that these sick infants cried more frequently than normal infants, and their mothers responded more quickly. The evolutionary significance of this is speculative, but exciting. Infants who perhaps need more protection elicit behaviors that intensify the protection response. The question of infant behavior as an elicitor of the maternal attachment response needs much more study in relation to high-risk infants.

GROWTH-FOSTERING ENVIRONMENTS

All parents want to provide the best environment possible for their children. The perplexing question has been: what is a growth-fostering environment? Any answer is contingent on understanding what outcomes are expected. Immediately, the issue of culture needs to be considered. In this review, the emphasis was on white middle-class culture since the majority of studies were done on that segment. In the white middle-class culture, there is a value on intelligence and on the child's growing up to become socially and economically independent of the family of origin. There is an expectation that the child will become increasingly skilled with language and will be able to communicate effectively with others. While there are few clear expectations about social behavior, excessive aggression, hostility, and depression are not generally viewed as desirable.

The Nursing Child Assessment Project (NCAP) was undertaken by Barnard and Douglas in 1974 to identify what early factors about the child and environment were related to later developmental problems. Measures of the child, parent, and parent-child interaction were developed and/or adapted (Barnard & Eyres, 1979; Eyres, Barnard, & Gray, Note 5). A sample of 193 first-born newborns and their families was studied. The sample was stratified for equal representation of low and high risk as well as high and low maternal education. Subjects were studied during the first four years of life, and 87 percent of the children were followed until the fourth year of life. This constituted one of the largest and most comprehensive studies of young children and their environment in the recent decades. The study had both descriptive and methodological goals. The descriptive purpose was to identify factors from the earliest period of life, pregnancy, and the first two years that were related to the child's later developmental status. The major findings were that: (a) measures of perinatal or infant physical status were extremely weak predictors of IQ or language at 4 years of age; (b) assessments of mother-infant interaction and general environmental quality were among the best predictors at each age tested and were as good as measures of child performance at 24 and 36 months in predicting IQ and language; (c) assessments of child performance were poor predictors prior to 24 months but excellent predictors of later status from 24 months on; (d) measures of family ecology (levels of stress, social support, maternal education) and parent perception of the child, especially when assessed at birth, were strongly related to child IQ and language within the low education subsample, but not among mothers with more than high school education (Bee, Barnard, Eyres, Gray, Hammond, Spietz, Snyder, & Clark, 1982).

One of the most widely used measures of the growth-fostering environment of children from birth to 3 years is the Home Observation for Measuring the Environment (HOME), developed by Caldwell and colleagues (Bradley & Caldwell, 1976, 1980). There are six subscales, including emotional and verbal responsivity of the mother, avoidance of restriction and punishment, organization of the environment, provision of appropriate play materials, and opportunities for variety in daily stimulation. The total HOME score is correlated positively with later mental development and is a better predictor of the later mental status than are measures of the child's mental development under the age of 2 years.

In a recent analysis of the Seattle NCAP sample, with HOME inventory scores from the first three years of life, Barnard, Bee, and Hammond (in press) replicated the Bradley and Caldwell (1980) finding that there are age-specific aspects of the environment that appear to show significant relationships with later IQ. For instance, the subscales Maternal Involvement and Variety of Stimulation appeared to be important at 8 to 12 months, while Level of Restriction and Punishment appeared particularly relevant at 24 months (Barnard, Bee, & Hammond, in press). Such findings, when further replicated, will have obvious implications for nursing intervention; they will give guidance to where the focus should be in helping the parents provide a growth-fostering environment. There is also the need to raise new questions. What encourages a parent to be restrictive? What factors are associated with maternal involvement and responsiveness? Barnard (1981) reported that maternal involvement was correlated with the mother's report of whether her needs for emotional support were met, and the tendency to be restrictive was correlated positively with maternal education and the child's activity level. While these parental qualities were correlated positively, there clearly were four patterns: involved-nonrestrictive; involved-restrictive; less involved-nonrestrictive; and less involved-restrictive. These four typologies would be a potential measure of parental styles in future research about the early childrearing environment.

Negative Environments

The opposite question—what environments do not foster growth?—can be studied with abused, neglected, and failure-to-thrive children. The scenario by and large suggests limited parent-child interaction and a high use of negative responses. Child abuse involves more active aggression toward the child, while in neglect and failure-to-thrive cases, the parent is more passive and fails to provide interaction, stimulation, or physical care (Parks, 1978; Corey, Miller & Widlak, 1975).

Westra and Martin (1981) reported a study of the children of abused mothers. They found these children demonstrated more aggression than other children, impaired cognitive abilities, delays in verbal development, and poor motor abilities. The authors suggested that the children may be affected by the altered family structure and function and acquire patterns of behavior through observing the passivity of the mother and aggression of the father. Alternatively, they proposed that children inhibit autonomous ego functions such as language, learning, or motor skills when faced with an externally dangerous environment.

Durand (1975) gave a comprehensive review of the problem of failure to thrive and maternal deprivation. She presented a case study of a 5-year-old Down's syndrome child with "masked" maternal deprivation. The importance of this work is both the theoretical clarity brought to the problem and the model presented for nursing diagnosis and treatment. During a 17-day period of nursing care designed to provide both structure and contingent stimulation for the child, there was a remarkable gain in length and weight, increased sleep, increased awareness of the environment, and less self-stimulating behavior. In spite of less caloric intake during the period of planned nursing care compared to the prior intake, the child showed physical growth. This study demonstrated the fact that the growth-fostering environment must be one that matches the child's developmental need and sensory capacity for processing stimulation. In this case, the nonmatch was central to the "masked" deprivation. Observations of the mother's care revealed that in spite of a stimulating and caring approach to the child, there was little evidence that maternal activities were responsive to the child's behavior and capacity to assimilate.

In addition to the general qualities of stimulation described to be of importance, such as variety, complexity, and responsiveness (Yarrow, Rubinstein, & Pedersen, 1975), the examination of the negative growth-fostering environments revealed that an essential part of providing a growth-fostering environment is the mediation provided by the adult caregiver. This mediation involves protecting the child from too much input, matching the input to status of readiness, and modifying the stimulation to the responsiveness of the child.

The adult's role as a mediator for the child involves the development of a communication system between the adult and the child. In recent studies, investigators have reported methods of rating this parent-child interaction. In the NCAP (Barnard & Eyres, 1979), two observational scales were developed to measure parent-child interaction. One observation was structured around the familiar feeding situation; the mother's sensitivity and adaptability were scored on 11 items, and the infant's adaptability and responsiveness to the mother were scored on 10 separate items. The second observation was made during an episode where the mother was asked to teach her infant a task, such as to reach for a red ring, or to stack blocks, depending on the child's age. The resulting maternal cluster scores measured maternal positive messages, negative messages, task facilitation, and instructional techniques. The infant's cluster was readiness to learn. The psychometrics of the scales were reported in Barnard and Eyres (1979). There was acceptable internal consistency of the constructs and moderate long-term test-retest reliability. The major problem was training and obtaining high interobserver correlations.

Revision of the scales was accomplished by converting the scaling from a five-point interval scale for teaching and a seven-point interval scale for feeding to a binary yes or no option. The thematic content was also restructured to lend itself to a presence or absence scoring. The construct used in the revisions to characterize the parent-child interactive process was one in which the central themes were the sensitivity and responsiveness of the dyad. The construct which described the parental behavior was composed of sensitivity to cues, response to distress, and providing both a social-emotional growth-fostering and a cognitive growth-fostering environment. The child's behavior consisted of clarity of cues and responsiveness to the parent. The revised version has not been used in any predictive studies to date. However, the total scale scores do differentiate groups where there is a suspected or actual parent-child problem, such as child abuse, failure-to-thrive, premature infants, low education mothers (Barnard & Bee, in press).

Thus the evidence suggests that good communication between parents and young children is important for fostering development. Good communication is characterized by each member of the dyad's being active in the communication and responsive to the other partner. The parents' role, however, extends beyond the process of communication and involves the information the parent communicates, such as affection, approval or disapproval, and features of the environment.

HOSPITALIZATION

The studies involving hospitalized children have centered largely on the child's reaction to the hospitalization or to the procedure involved. The literature implies that children are more vulnerable because they are younger and have less ability to comprehend what is happening. Three descriptive studies that present many issues for further study about separation and parental care are discussed here.

Children's Reactions to Hospitalization

Parental rooming-in was the focus of Fletcher's work (1981). Fletcher hypothesized that the child from 6 months to 3 years of age is particularly influenced by the separation from this attachment figure, since this is the period of development when the child is learning whom he can depend on to meet his needs. Fletcher asked how the child reacts to the mother who is rooming-in during the period of hospitalization. Utilizing a single case study design, he investigated the avoidance, approach, and reactive behaviors of a 20-month-old child hospitalized for repair of a hypospadias.

The results of this observational study over a 9-day period, including one day of preoperative data and seven days of postoperative data, documented the occurrence of all three behaviors. There was a striking number of avoidance behaviors following surgery, in contrast to the preoperative period, when there were none. How could this be explained, when the avoidance behavior, commonly described as the denial stage for children showing separation response, occurred in a child whose mother was present?

Fletcher posed alternative explanations: the child was uncertain if the mother would respond to meet his needs in this strange situation, so he avoided the dependence; the child had previous feelings of ambivalence which were increased with this experience, hence the avoidance; the child saw his mother as less predictable since she was not eliminating his distress and may actually have let this hurt come to him; the mother was uncertain and frustrated and did not behave in the usual sensitive manner, thus increasing the child's distress.

It is appropriate to raise yet another line of reasoning. Perhaps the surgery resulted in both a physiological and a psychological disorganization. This state of system disorganization would be accompanied by an inability to deal with incoming stimuli; the avoidance, therefore, might be a regulatory behavior on the part of the child, seeking to reduce an overload to the system.

My own past research with premature infants (Barnard, 1972; Barnard & Bee, in press) leads me to propose that when the organism is unstable, there is a reduced capacity to deal with incoming stimuli. Prematures shut out stimuli during feeding; typically they have their eyes closed or turn their heads away from the feeding for frequent and prolonged intervals. This behavior gradually subsides and is less prominent after 4 months. It seems reasonable to ask how system disorganization in hospitalized children may influence their avoidance, approach, and reaction behavior. Researchers need to know more about what aspects of caregiving prevent disorganization or re-regulate the system. Perhaps by experiencing a regular sequence and timing of care, the unstable individual would use the structure provided by the care to restore system regulation. A study in which the time of feedings, positioning, or maternal contact is carefully structured to occur at regular intervals rather than spontaneously would be an appropriate way to begin testing this proposition.

Almost no data exist at present on the reaction to hospitalizaton of the infant under 6 months of age; acceptance of the age specificity (6 to 36 months) of attachment has discouraged such investigation. Yet we know from studies with well, term infants that caregiver behavior has an influence on sleep and crying (Sander, Stechler, Burns, & Lee, 1979; Youngberg, 1978). In a study under way in Sweden, a nurse investigator (Elander, Note 6) is examining the behavioral, physiological, and biochemical responses of infants under 6 months when cared for by mother, by other caregivers, and also when hospitalized. Thus, two expansions seem in order relating to questions about the hospitalization of young children: (a) the role that system organization or disorganization plays in the child's response to the caregiver and to hospitalization, and (b) the enlargement of how the child under 6 months of age expresses reaction to separation and the loss of the previous environmental patterning.

Children's Reactions to Procedures

In a study on releasing the hospitalized child from restraints, Dowd, Novak, and Ray, (1977) included 29 children and demonstrated a more specific focus of investigation into the care practices used to accommodate the treatment needs of the hospitalized child. Restraints are frequently used in pediatric nursing to prevent the child from dislodging tubing and/or doing harm to an irritated body part or site. Increasingly complicated medical regimes, requiring life-support systems and other technological gadgets for monitoring and treatment, make it likely that restraints are an increasing issue in the care of hospitalized children. Dowd et al. (1977) put forth assumptions about the individual's need for motor activity. They cited both physiological and behavioral evidence concerning the effects of restricting mobility. They concluded that mobility is essential for maintaining the integrity of the physiological function of all body systems and for promoting normal motor and psychosocial skills. From this conceptual framework, they sought to study how children who required restraints would respond when the restraints were temporarily removed. These investigators found that there was an age differential in response to being freed. Children under 18 months were observed to cry and fight their restraints, and when freed the infants were initially immobile. Only as the restraints were repeatedly removed did the activity levels and protest behaviors against being restrained again increase. The older children tended to protest the restraints less vigorously, and when the restraints were removed they had no generalizable response. Over time their protest to the reapplication of restraints diminished; it was as if they had learned that the nurse would return and give them freedom. The important observation was that neither infants nor older children made any attempt to disturb tubes or sutures.

This study generates many questions for further study. For example, can some initial, intermittent restraint teach a child not to bother certain tubes or bandages? One version of the treatment could be both verbal explanation of the desired behavior and restraint when the child behaved undesirably, and no restraint when the desirable behavior was present. For children with a definite need for restraint, the practice of regular, supervised episodes free from restraint would be the basis for an experiment. A design could be set up in which the independent variable would be intermittent free mobility and the dependent variables could be metabolic function as measured in the excretion of essential electrolytes known to be altered by immobilization, or the child's avoidance, approach, and reactive behaviors.

Hagemann (1981a, 1981b) presented an important finding about the amount of sleep that preschool children got when hospitalized and how much their sleep was disrupted. The majority of sleep disruption was from external stimuli, such as noise and caretaking. From the sample of thirty-four children observed throughout the night following their admission, only four children did not have their sleep interrupted. Forty-two out of 118 disruptions were for assessment of vital signs. The mean number of disruptions per child, including external as well as internal, was 3.47. This study demonstrated that sleep of hospitalized infants and children was affected by the nursing care and that nursing care needs to be altered to minimize the impact. Children with either a history of previous hospital admission or whose present hospital admission was for medical conditions were more often aroused from internal causes such as physiological and psychological discomfort. Certainly much more study needs to be done with improvement of the methods used to observe sleep and with observing the relationship between sleep deprivation and well-being.

Many treatments are given to children in the hospital: intrusive procedures such as injections, catheterizations, and oxygen administration. Very little research has been conducted on how the developmental stage and the personal life history of the child influence the response to these treatments. Many of the studies that have been done are case studies; the potential value of knowledge that can be generalized will be lost if the insights from these small samples are not carried to further descriptive large samples and, when appropriate, to clinical trials or true experiments.

The young child's response to hospitalization has been studied by both nurses and members of other disciplines (Fletcher, 1981; Robertson, 1970). The knowledge available provides general information to researchers. It is known that the child from 6 to 36 months is especially vulnerable to separation. It is known that children have a smoother recovery when the parent remains with the child. There is not sufficient data on the responses of the infant under 6 months of age. There are no data about how previous separations influence the child's response to separation. There is very little literature dealing with specific events and experiences based on the child's age or condition. A great deal can be learned from studying the experience and caregiving of hospitalized children that can both improve care and promote recovery and growth.

SUMMARY, RESEARCH DIRECTIONS

Nursing research concerning infants and young children relative to four specific health issues, prematurity, attachment, growth-fostering environments, and hospitalization, was reviewed. Questions asked were about self-regulatory behavior of the preterm infant relative to immaturity and the external environment, about facilitating attachment of parents to children, and about factors associated with promoting the development of children. These investigations add to the empirical data base but as yet do not elaborate a more specific theoretical base for nursing science. The work being advanced on sucking as a self-regulating behavior should provide an important model for theory development. The investigations concerning environmental stimulation of premature infants provide a basis for returning to the theoretical notions about how external stimuli influence the function and development of the central nervous system; there is need to clarify whether the preterm infant needs arousing or soothing and whether external stimuli aid in self-regulation.

There is also need to redefine the theoretical assumptions about parental attachment. Clarification of attachment, what it is and how it develops, could improve the descriptive and experimental work of the future. Rubin's (1977) assumptions about binding-in are a logical starting point. Rubin assumed that reciprocity is largely accomplished by the end of pregnancy, yet most research in this area emphasized the need for reciprocity in the early postpartum period. Additional questions about how environmental circumstances influence parental attachment need to be formulated. For example, how does the relationship network of the parent influence parent-child attachment? When infants are hospitalized in the early months of life, what impact does this have on parent-child attachment? There is need for more descriptive work on parent-child attachment. Little is known about the process over time and how varying circumstances of the parent or child influence the process or outcomes.

In studies concerning growth-fostering characteristics of the child's environment, researchers have begun to identify factors, such as parent-child communication, parental styles, and general qualities of the home environment, that can now be used to examine how these same factors relate to differing cultural groups and child characteristics. Studies about the hospitalization experience need to move forward to answer new questions about what aspects of the hospital experience are disruptive to the child and how these episodes influence the child's behavior and recovery.

Along with specifying anew questions asked about children's responses to actual or potential health problems, there is evidence of need for methods to measure these responses. Suggestions were made throughout the chapter about needed measures.

REFERENCE NOTES

1. Anderson, G. C., Dahm, J., Ellis, M., & Vidyasagar, D. Effect of time-controlled sucking opportunities on sucking pressures and arousal in high-risk infants. Paper presented at the meeting of the American Nurses' Association, Council of Nurse Researchers, Washington, D.C., September 1981.
2. Barnard, K. E., & Bee, H. L. *Premature infant refocus. Final report*. Unpublished manuscript, 1981. (Available from University of Washington, School of Nursing, Seattle, Washington.)
3. Barnard, K. E., & Bee, H. L. The impact of temporally patterned stimulation on the development of preterm infants. Manuscript submitted for publication, 1982.
4. Price, G. M. *Maternal-infant adaptation scale*. Worcester, Massachusetts, 1975.
5. Eyres, S. J., Barnard, K. E., & Gray, C. A. *Child health assessment Part 3: 2–4 years*. Unpublished manuscript, 1979. (Available from University of Washington, School of Nursing, Seattle, Washington.)
6. Elander, G. University of Lund, Pediatric Institute, Malmo, Sweden. Personal communication, September 1982.

REFERENCES

Ainsworth, M. The development of infant-mother attachment. In B. L. Caldwell & H. Ricciuti (Eds.), *Review of child development research* (Vol. 3). Chicago: University of Chicago Press, 1973.
American Nurses' Association. *Nursing, a social policy statement*. Kansas City, Missouri: American Nurses' Association, 1981.
Anderson, C. Enhancing reciprocity between mother and neonate. *Nursing Research*, 1981, *30*, 89–93.

Anderson, G. C., & Vidyasagar, D. Development of sucking in premature infants from 1 to 7 days postbirth. In G. C. Anderson & B. Raff (Eds.), *Newborn behavioral organization: Nursing research and implications* (Vol. 15). New York: Alan R. Liss, 1979.

Barnard, K. E. The effect of stimulation on the duration of sleep and wakefulness in the premature infant (Doctoral dissertation, University of Washington, 1972). *Dissertation Abstracts International,* 1972, *33,* 2167B. (University Microfilms No. 72-28573)

Barnard, K. E. General issues in parent-infant interaction during the first years of life. In D. L. Yeung (Ed.), *Essays on pediatric nutrition.* Ontario, Canada: The Canadian Science Committee on Food and Nutrition, Canadian Public Health Association, 1981.

Barnard, K. E., & Bee, H. L. The assessment of parent-infant interaction by observation of feeding and teaching. In T. B. Brazelton & H. Als (Eds.), *New approaches to developmental screening of infants.* New York: Elsevier North Holland, in press.

Barnard, K. E., Bee, H. L., & Hammond, M. A. Home environment in a healthy low risk sample: The Seattle study. In A. W. Gottfried (Ed.), *Home environment and early mental development.* New York: Academic Press, in press.

Barnard, K. E., & Douglas, H. B. (Eds.). *Child health assessment Part 1. A literature review.* Dept. of Health, Education, & Welfare, Pub. No. (HRA) 75-30, Stock No. 1741-00081. Washington, D.C.: Government Printing Office, 1974.

Barnard, K. E., & Eyres, S. J. (Eds.). *Child health assessment Part 2. The first year of life.* Dept. of Health, Education, & Welfare, Pub. No. (HRA) 79-25, Stock No. 017-041-00131-9. Washington, D.C.: Government Printing Office, 1979.

Bee, H. L., Barnard, K. E., Eyres, S. J., Gray, C. A., Hammond, M. A., Spietz, A. L., Snyder, C., & Clark, B. Prediction of IQ and language skill from perinatal status, child performance, family characteristics, and mother-infant interaction. *Child Development,* 1982, *53,* 1134-1156.

Bowlby, J. *Attachment and loss* (Vol. 1), *Attachment.* New York: Basic Books, 1969.

Bradley, R. H., & Caldwell, B. M. Early home environment and changes in mental test performance in children from 6 to 36 months. *Developmental Psychology,* 1976, *12,* 93-97.

Bradley, R. H., & Caldwell, B. M. The relation of home environment, cognitive competence and IQ among males and females. *Child Development,* 1980, *51,* 1140-1148.

Brazelton, T. B. *Neonatal behavioral assessment scale.* Philadelphia: J. B. Lippincott, 1973.

Carter-Jessop, L. Promoting maternal attachment through prenatal intervention. *MCN, American Journal of Maternal Child Nursing,* 1981, *6,* 107-112.

Casler, L. Maternal deprivation: A critical review of the literature. *Monographs of the Society for Research in Child Development,* 1961, *26,* 1-64.

Chapman, J. S. The relationship between auditory stimulation and gross motor activity of short-gestation infants. *Research in Nursing and Health,* 1978, *1,* 29-36.

Chapman, J. S. Influence of varied stimuli on development of motor patterns in the premature infant. In G. C. Anderson & B. Raff (Eds.), *Newborn behavioral organization: Nursing research and implications* (Vol. 15). New York: Alan R. Liss, 1979.

Collins, J. E. Cardiac responses during mechanical ventilation of neonates with respiratory distress syndrome. *Journal of Advanced Nursing*, 1978, *3*, 73–83.

Corey, E. J. B., Miller, C. L., & Widlak, F. W. Factors contributing to child abuse. *Nursing Research*, 1975, *24*, 293–295.

Cranley, M. S. Development of a tool for the measurement of maternal attachment during pregnancy. *Nursing Research*, 1981, *30*, 281–284.

Curry, M. A. Maternal attachment behavior and the mother's self-concept: The effect of early skin-to-skin contact. *Nursing Research*, 1982, *31*, 73–77.

De Chateau, P. Neonatal care routines: Influences on maternal and infant behavior and on breastfeeding. (Unpublished doctoral dissertation, Umea University, Umea, Sweden, 1976.)

Dowd, E. L., Novak, J. C., & Ray, E. J. Releasing the hospitalized child from restraints. *MCN, American Journal of Maternal Child Nursing*, 1977, *2*, 370–373.

Durand, B. A clincal nursing study: Failure to thrive in a child with Down's syndrome. *Nursing Research*, 1975, *24*, 272–286.

Ellison, S. E., Vidyasagar, D., & Anderson, G. C. Sucking in the newborn infant during the first hour of life. *Journal of Nurse-Midwifery*, 1979, *24*, 18–25.

Fletcher, B. Rooming-in: A reassessment. *Maternal-Child Nursing Journal*, 1981, *10*, 85–97.

Hagemann, V. Night sleep of children in hospital. Part I. Sleep duration. *Maternal-Child Nursing Journal*, 1981, *10*, 1–14. (a)

Hagemann, V. Night sleep of children in hospital. Part II. Sleep disruption. *Maternal-Child Nursing Journal*, 1981, *10*, 127–141. (b)

Holaday, B. Maternal response to their chronically ill infants' attachment behavior of crying. *Nursing Research*, 1981, *30*, 343–348.

Holaday, B. Maternal conceptual set development: Identifying patterns of maternal response to chronically ill infant crying. *Maternal-Child Nursing Journal*, 1982, *11*, 47–59.

Jones, C. Father to infant attachment: Effects of early contact and characteristics of the infant. *Research in Nursing and Health*, 1981, *4*, 193–200.

Kang, R. The relationship between informing both parents of their infant's behavioral response patterns and the mother's perception of the infant. (Unpublished master's thesis, University of Washington, 1974.)

Klaus, M. H., Jerauld, R. N., Kreger, N. C., McAlpine, W., Steffa, M., & Kennell, J. H. Maternal attachment, importance of the first post-partum days. *New England Journal of Medicine*, 1972, *286*, 460–463.

Klaus, M. H., & Kennell, J. H. Mothers separated from their newborns. *Pediatric Clinics of North America*, 1970, *17*, 1015–1037.

Kramer, M., Chamorro, I., Green, D., & Knudtson, F. Extra tactile stimulation of the premature infant. *Nuring Research*, 1975, *24*, 324–334.

Malloy, G. The relationship between maternal and musical auditory stimulation and the developmental behavior of premature infants. In G. C. Anderson & B. Raff (Eds.), *Newborn behavioral organization: Nursing research and implications* (Vol. 15). New York: Alan R. Liss, 1979.

Measal, C. P., & Anderson, G. C. Nonnutritive sucking during tube feedings: Effect on clinical course in premature infants. *Journal of Obstetric, Gynecologic and Neonatal Nursing*, 1979, *8*, 265–272.

Neal, M. V. Organization behavior of the premature infant. In G. C. Anderson & B. Raff (Eds.), *Newborn behavioral organization: Nursing research and implications* (Vol. 15). New York: Alan R. Liss, 1979.

Pannabecker, B. J., & Emde, R. N. The effect of extended contact on father-newborn interaction. In M. V. Batey (Ed.), *Communicating nursing research* (Vol. 10). Boulder, Colo.: Western Interstate Commission for Higher Education, 1977.

Parks, K. M. Failure to thrive as a result of maternal deprivation. *Current Practice Obstetrics and Gynecological Nursing*, 1978, *2*, 190–196.

Rausch, P. D. Effects of tactile and kinesthetic stimulation on premature infants. *Journal of Obstetric, Gynecologic and Neonatal Nursing*, 1981, *10*, 34–37.

Rice, R. The effects of the Rice infant sensorimotor stimulation treatment on the development of high-risk infants. In G. C. Anderson & B. Raff (Eds.), *Newborn behavioral organization: Nursing research and implications* (Vol. 15). New York: Alan R. Liss, 1979.

Robertson, J. *Young children in hospitals*. New York: Barnes and Noble, 1970.

Rubin, R. Binding-in in the postpartum period. *Maternal-Child Nursing Journal*, 1977, *6*, 67–75.

Ryan, L. Maternal perception of neonatal behavior. (Unpublished master's thesis, University of Washington, School of Nursing, 1973.)

Sander, L. W., Stechler, C., Burns, P., & Lee, A. Change in infant and caregiver variables over the first two months of life: Integration of action in early development. In E. B. Thoman (Ed.), *Origins of infant's social responsiveness*. Hillsdale, N. J.: Lawrence Erlbaum, 1979.

Spitz, R. A. Anxiety in infants. *International Journal of Psychoanalysis*, 1950, *31*, 138–143.

Westra, B., & Martin, H. P. Children of battered women. *Maternal-Child Nursing Journal*, 1981, *10*, 41–54.

Yarrow, L. J. Rubenstein, J. L., & Pedersen, F. A. *Infant and environment, early cognitive and motivational development*. Washington, D. C.: Hemisphere, 1975.

Youngberg, S. L. P. The effect of cycled and uncycled lighting on the sleep behavior of neonates (Doctoral dissertation, University of Washington, 1978.) *Dissertation Abstracts International*, 1978, *39*, 2550B. (University Microfilms No. 78–20791)

CHAPTER 2

Nursing Research Related to Schoolage Children and Adolescents

MARY J. DENYES
COLLEGE OF NURSING
WAYNE STATE UNIVERSITY

CONTENTS

The review of nursing research in this chapter includes studies published between 1952 and early 1982. Investigations pertaining to children and adolescents between the ages of 6 and 18 years that were reported in major nursing research journals or maternal child nursing journals are included. Additionally, the review includes nursing studies reported in other nurs-

27

ing journals or journals of other disciplines and retrieved by computer searches, search of nursing indexes, review of reference lists of related studies, or informal contacts of the author. While these search techniques yielded a large number of studies for review, the limitations in formal indexing of nursing publications may have left relevant research unidentified.

Research reported within the context of the nursing practice setting and related to the child/adolescent, the nurse, or the interaction of the two is reviewed. Relevant studies included in other chapters of the *Annual Review of Nursing Research* (e.g., studies of parents and families of schoolage children or adolescent pregnancy) are not reviewed here.

The organization of the chapter was approached inductively. Major concepts and themes in the studies were identified and used as organizing schema. The three main areas of inquiry that evolved were: (a) child and adolescent perceptions of self, life events, and environment; (b) child and adolescent responses to self, life events, and environment; and (c) therapeutic nursing interventions with children and adolescents. The concepts of health, illness, stress, health promotion, health care, and hospitalization were ones that recurred throughout these three main areas of inquiry.

The studies are clustered conceptually. Major findings are reviewed. Major strengths and limitations are identified with respect to conceptualization, methods, and potential for generation of knowledge that is practice-relevant. A general critique and recommendations for strengthening the knowledge base for nursing practice with children and adolescents are provided at the conclusion of the chapter.

CHILD AND ADOLESCENT PERCEPTIONS

Perceptions of Self

Knowledge generated through nursing studies relative to child and adolescent perceptions of self, life events, and environment was limited. Areas of inquiry related to perceptions of self included study of children's knowledge of their bodies, capabilities for self-care, and self-concepts and identities.

Porter (1974), Quiggin (1977), and Williams (1978) examined children's perceptions of their internal body parts. Schoolage children were asked to draw on body outlines everything inside their bodies and to name those body parts. Quiggin and Williams also interviewed the children about their understanding of body functions. The researchers found that chil- dren's knowledge of their bodies was relatively extensive and accurate in terms of structure, position, and function. Additional findings were that the quality and quantity of knowledge varied with age (Porter, 1974). Boys at all ages identified more body parts than did girls (Porter, 1974; Quiggin, 1977). Both well and hospitalized American children had significantly higher body organ scores than did respective groups of Filipino children (Williams, 1978). Although constituted by convenience, the samples in- cluded well and hospitalized children ranging in age from 6 to 11 years drawn from populations in the United States ($N = 144, 146$), England ($N = 46$), and the Philippines ($N = 166$).

Three particular strengths of these studies of children's perceptions of internal body parts were noted. The first was that Quiggin's (1977) work built directly upon the previous nursing research of Porter (1974). There were relatively few instances found in this literature review in which the researcher carefully designed a study to take into account and build upon prior nursing research. While Williams (1978) did not draw upon the Porter or Quiggin work, she did present a comparison of data from two previously unpublished or relatively inaccessible sources. A second strength, especial- ly with respect to the Quiggin and Porter studies, was that they provided a good beginning data base for health teaching with children. An understand- ing of the extent and accuracy of children's knowledge of their bodies is an important component in planning nursing interventions designed to assist children relative to health promotion. A third strength was the yield of data about similarities and differences in perceptions of children from different cultural groups.

A second area of inquiry about child and adolescent perceptions of self was capabilities of self-care. While a number of nurse researchers have addressed the concept of self-care (Denyes, 1982; Lewis, C. E., Lewis, M. A., Lorimer, & Palmer, 1977; Pridham, 1971), Denyes (1982) focused on client perceptions of self. This research involved the development of a self-report questionnaire to measure adolescent capability for self-care (self-care agency). A sample of 161 adolescents aged 14 to 18 years was used; the population from which the sample was drawn was not specified. The procedures used for instrument development and initial reliability and validity testing were reported. The strength of this study lay in the apparent- ly sound theoretical and methodological base of the instrument develop- ment and in its potential use in both nursing practice and research.

Benoliel (1970) explored events and experiences that contribute to development of one's perception of self as a diabetic. A theoretical sample of nine families containing thirteen youths with diabetes was selected for study. Specific examination of the findings was precluded by the very limited data presented.

Collectively, the nursing studies related to child and adolescent perception of self provided a meager but real beginning knowledge base. Data regarding youths' knowledge of their bodies, a means of measuring perceived self-care capabilities, and glimpses of self-perception among youth with chronic illness were generated.

Perceptions of Life Events and Environment

Nursing studies of child and adolescent perceptions of life events and environment included exploration of death (Swain, 1979), illness (Brodie, 1974; Williams, 1978), and locus of control (Eggland, 1973). In her interviews with 120 healthy children from 2 to 16 years of age, Swain found that concepts of death differed by age with respect to finality, inevitability, and acknowledgment of death as a personal event. No differences were found among children of differing educational or religious backgrounds. Strengths of the research included attention to interrater reliability, appropriate data analysis, and clear presentation of data. In the Brodie (1974) study, analysis of questionnaire data on illness and anxiety from 408 first, third, and fifth graders revealed that healthy, nonanxious youth rejected views that illness was a punishment, evoked a negative response from parents, and was disruptive to their lives. Anxious children perceived illness in these negative ways. While useful new data were generated, the investigator moved beyond the reported data in the conclusions. Williams (1978) studied knowledge of illness in well and hospitalized third and fifth graders in two countries. No significant differences were found between American and Filipino youth. Knowledge levels were not influenced by demographic variables. Appropriate, though not sophisticated analyses were done. Relevance to nursing was not addressed in any of these three studies.

Eggland (1973) compared locus of control in two groups of schoolage children. Twenty first and fourth graders with cerebral palsy perceived life events to result from external forces to a greater degree than did the 82 children of the same age who had no physical disability. Gender differences were not significant. Eggland drew upon previous empirical and theoretical work and used a valid, reliable instrument. The investigator's decision not to obtain informed consent for the children with cerebral palsy was of concern.

This cluster of studies related to child and adolescent perceptions of life events and environment provided a fragmented initial data base. Knowledge about healthy children's conceptions of death, and healthy and ill children's perceptions of illness and locus of control was generated.

CHILD AND ADOLESCENT RESPONSES

Responses to General Life Events and Environment

Personal, family, and social life change events believed to be stressful to adolescents were examined by several nurse researchers (Beard, 1980; Mendez, Yeaworth, York, & Goodwin, 1980; Yeaworth, York, Hussey, Ingle, & Goodwin, 1980). Building upon earlier work with adults, Mendez et al (1980) and Yeaworth et al. (1980) developed and refined an instrument to measure the amount of stress adolescents perceived resulting from each of a series of life change events. Two convenience samples of 11- to 18-year-old youths from white, middle, upper-middle, and upper socioeconomic classes were studied ($N = 207$; 182). While limited attention was given to instrument reliability and validity, adolescents, like adults in previous studies, rated death and separation as most stressful. Reported differences between adolescents of differing socioeconomic classes were difficult to interpret because of methodological inconsistencies.

In her study of interpersonal trust, life events, and coping in 94 black youths from 13 to 18 years of age, Beard (1980) found coping and life events were related, but found no relationship between trust and life events, or between trust and coping. Conceptualization and relevance to nursing were clearly presented; interpretation of findings was limited by inconsistencies in reporting of the analyses.

Investigators in the other nursing studies of responses to general life events and environment addressed childhood fears and responses to violence, change in family residence, and parental disability. A small cluster of research was conducted on childhood fears. Astin (1977) found that political, natural, and ecological phenomena were the fear categories mentioned most by 10- to 12-year-old hospitalized ($N = 25$) and nonhospitalized ($N = 26$) youths. Fears of separation and death were prevalent. Although there were some differences in intensity of fears, there were no significant differences in number of fears between the two groups. There were no differences in average number reported by gender or race. The developmental framework for the study was clearly presented and consistent with other studies on childhood fears (Miller, 1979). Description of methods was extremely scant. Yanni (1982) hypothesized that fearfulness among 10- and 11-year-old females would be related to perception of parental support, punishment, control, and encouragement of autonomy, but found that these parental factors accounted for very little of the variance in the girls' fearfulness ($N = 68$). The research process was clearly described; the study would have been strengthened by more careful attention to its conceptual base.

Westra and Martin (1981) and Burgess and Holmstrom (1974) examined youths' responses to violence in their lives and environment. Twenty middle class, ethnically diverse boys and girls selected by convenience from shelters for battered women showed more aggression than other children, demonstrated delays in verbal development, and manifested impaired cognitive and motor abilities (Westra & Martin, 1981). The study was sound theoretically and methodologically. Although children and adolescents were included in the sample of rape victims interviewed by Burgess and Holmstrom (1974), their responses generally were not identified separately; thus examination of those responses was impossible.

Van Dongen (1981) examined attitudes toward family change in residence and postmove adjustment in 35 youths 6 to 12 years of age. She found no postmove behavioral change in the majority of the children; where change was noted, it was most often favorable. Children's attitudes toward moving did not reflect their parents' attitudes toward moving. There was little association between parental or children's attitudes toward moving and children's postmove adjustment, age, gender, distance moved, or reason for move. Strengths of the research included articulation with previous theoretical and empirical work and relevance of findings for anticipatory health guidance with families. Analysis appeared appropriate, although not all aspects were fully described.

In her study of responses to parental disability, Olgas (1974) found that children of parents with multiple sclerosis did not respond significantly differently on body image scales from children of healthy parents. The study was conceptualized clearly in terms of identification and was strengthened by a sampling plan that took into account gender of parents and children. Some differences in responses associated with gender were found. Conclusions drawn by the investigator did not differentiate clearly between findings that were statistically significant and those that were not.

The nursing research related to child and adolescent responses to general life events and environment included both small clusters of studies and single research efforts. The clusters yielded data and instrumentation for measuring adolescent responses to personal, family, and social change as well as descriptive data about childhood fears and responses to violence in the form of rape and physical abuse of their mothers. The single research efforts yielded data about children's behavioral responses to moving and to disability in a parent.

Chronic Health Problems

Child and adolescent responses to chronic health problems constituted a major area of inquiry. Based on content analysis of verbatim recordings of observations and interviews with five 10- to 14-year-old youths, Ritchie (1977a, 1977b, 1980) identified patterns of response to leg amputation. The predominant responses were adjustive (e.g., seeking detailed information but limiting the amount received). Affective responses (i.e., depression, fear, rejection, and hope or pride), although less frequent, were a major part of the response pattern. Conceptual, methodological, and practice-related aspects of the research were well addressed.

Nathan (1977) investigated the responses of 10- to 15-year-old girls to scoliosis and surgical correction of the deformity. She found that approximately half of the convenience sample of 25 girls drew or described themselves as having a spinal curvature; half did not acknowledge the curvature. Interpretation of Rorschach Ink Blots suggested there was less fear about bodily vulnerability, less helplessness and passivity, and less anxiety among the young women who drew and talked about the curvature than among those who did not. While significant differences also were reported in figure drawings between older and younger girls, questions about the validity of the measures made interpretation of age findings unclear.

Garlinghouse and Sharp (1968) found relatively strong self-concepts among 18 5- to 15-year-old children with hemophilia, but found no significant association between self-concept and number of bleeding episodes. A significant association was found between numbers of family stresses and bleeding episodes. Based on a carefully conducted analysis, the investigators concluded that the children's self-concept appeared to act as a buffer against a certain amount of stress, but when the stresses reached a certain point, they affected bleeding.

Instruments to assess 6- to 12-year-old youths' responses to cystic fibrosis were developed by Rodgers, Ferholt, and Cooper (1974). Parent interview, teacher questionnaire, and parent demographic questionnaire data were obtained on psychosocial adjustment of 20 children. The teacher and parent demographic data added little to that obtained on parent interview. Attention was given to feasibility and reliability of the parent interview; however the focus on determining a psychiatric diagnosis suggested a limitation of this study as nursing research.

Findings of Eggland (1973) and Holaday (1974) suggested that youths with chronic illnesses and handicapping conditions were more externally oriented than were their well peers. Social learning theory was used as a conceptual base for both studies; attribution theory and a nursing systems model were integrated in Holaday's work. Twenty first and fourth graders with cerebral palsy were more externally controlled than 82 children in the same grades without physical disability (Eggland, 1973). Twenty-four chronically ill youths aged 8 to 17 years attributed more outcomes to external forces than did well youths. The additional finding that children diagnosed as chronically ill from birth attributed both success and failure to ability rather than to effort strengthened the sense that these youths did not perceive themselves to be in control of their lives (Holaday, 1974).

Hospitalization

Child and adolescent responses to hospitalization constituted another major area of inquiry. Patterns of response associated with different phases of hospitalization were identified by Savedra and Tesler (1981), Tesler and Savedra (1981), and Kueffner (1975). Savedra and Tesler studied 33 6- to 12-year-old children admitted to the hospital for elective surgery. They found that precoping or orienting responses accompanied the preoperative period, while behaviors designed to regulate or control surrounding stimuli predominated in the postoperative period. Few verbal, crying, or resistive behaviors were evidenced either before or after surgery. Limited differences by gender were found; no differences were associated with other demographic variables. There was evidence of reliability, validity, and conceptual consistency in the instruments developed and adapted to measure child and parent responses.

Kueffner (1975) found that six schoolage children hospitalized for treatment of severe burns progressed through stages of agony, hope, and reorganization. The first response stage, agony, lasted from entry into the hospital until the children sensed they had improved and would survive; it was characterized by a focus on self and pain. From that point until a discharge date was set, the response pattern was one of hope; responses reflected engagement with the environment. Responses during the final stage, reorganization, reflected concern with changes in body image and anticipated posthospital experiences; this stage ended with the children's actual discharge from hospital. Aloneness, pain, and loss were identified by Kueffner as major themes in the youths' responses to burns and isolation.

Fears of death, mutilation, pain, and abandonment were identified by Stoll (1969) in a study of three schoolage girls hospitalized for treatment of severe burns. Descriptive data were obtained for both the Kueffner and the Stoll studies by participant observation with small convenience samples of children 5 to 10 years of age. Kueffner included a careful description of the research process; that was missing from Stoll's work. Kueffner's research was an excellent example of the interface of research, practice, and theory building in nursing. Clinical data were observed, recorded, analyzed, interpreted, and organized carefully into a conceptual schema. Although gleaned from small convenience samples, detailed behavioral data regarding the experience of children who were burned, isolated, in pain, and undergoing changes in body image were generated. Questions to direct future research were identified.

Advances in knowledge of responses to hospitalization are dependent, in part, on the adequacy of the measurement instruments developed to describe those responses. Savedra and Tesler (1981) carefully addressed instrument development. Weiss (1969) developed a tool to summarize behavioral responses of youth in residential psychiatric settings. The Weiss instrument was comprised of a list of specific operationally defined behaviors used by nurses in practice (e.g., sleep irregularities, enuresis, barricading). A copy of the instrument was included in the report, but limited information about the development process was reported. Potential reliability testing was discussed, but not undertaken by the investigator.

Responses related to sleep and levels of consciousness in hospitalized youths were studied respectively by Hagemann (1981a, 1981b) and Barnes (1975). In her descriptive study of 34 children aged 3 to 8 years, Hagemann found sleep duration was 20 to 25 percent less during the first night in the hospital than it usually was at home, and that continuity of sleep was disrupted to some degree for all youths. Children's responses were recorded in categories of sleep, wakefulness, or arousal every five minutes throughout the night; environmental events also were recorded. The basic descriptive data on duration, onset, and termination of sleep, and on cause, frequency, and duration of sleep disruption were presented clearly and provided valuable direction for nursing practice and research. The statistical analyses and findings regarding relationships among many of the study variables were not reported clearly.

Predominant responses to intensive care unit phenomena (e.g., treatments, persons, equipment) among 13 youths aged 6 to 13 years were ones that showed alertness, awareness, and accuracy (Barnes, 1975). Motor and verbal responses identified from observation, drawing, and interview data were categorized into five levels of consciousness, including alertness, distortion, fantasy, affective memory, and dreams. Over half of the responses were categorized as alert, one-third were distorted; fantasy, affective memory, and dream responses were infrequent. Inclusion of the child's perception of the experience was a strength of the study.

Adolescent responses during hospitalization were studied by Daubenmire, Pierce, and Weaver (1960) and by Craft (1981). Data from graduate student logs suggested that 29 youths aged 12 to 21 years admitted to being ill and were aware of adjustments required by illness, but lacked inquisitiveness about their illnesses and accepted nurses and doctors as authority figures and information sources (Daubenmire et al., 1960). The absence of any description of data analysis made the interpretation of these findings difficult. In Craft's (1981) study, when 40 youths aged 12 to 17 years were offered a choice of a health professional, a parent, or both as information providers, health professionals were chosen most frequently. Additional findings about relationships between information provider preference and other variables were reported. However, errors in statistical analyses precluded conclusions being drawn from those data. Attention to the ways clients' preferences for information providers could be obtained and used in practice was a strength of the study.

Changes in self-esteem from admission to one month after admission were compared for three groups of youths aged 9 to 12 years (Riffee, 1981). Self-esteem in 25 youths hospitalized for surgery declined significantly more than in the 26 hospitalized for nonsurgical reasons and in the 28 nonhospitalized youths. Detailed description of all aspects of the research process, use of random sampling procedures, and careful attention to the interface with theory and practice were particular strengths of Riffee's work.

Health Care Procedures

Areas of inquiry related to youths' responses to health care procedures included response to hemodialyis (Neff, 1978), medical diagnostic procedures (Mandleco, 1976; Youssef, 1981), surgery (Barnes, 1969), binocular bandages (Riddle, 1972), immunizations (Hester, 1979), and physical examination (Mitchell, 1980). Neff's data, derived from observations and interviews with five youths aged 10 to 15 years, revealed three major types of responses to hemodialysis. They were, in order of frequency of occurrence: orienting, resistive, and adaptive. Bodily function changes constituted the major content of the responses. Orienting responses also were prevalent among ten 7- to 11-year-old children experiencing hospital admission and nonintrusive cardiac diagnostic procedures (Youssef, 1981). Responses reflecting a loss of control were seen in those youths only during the intrusive procedure of cardiac catheterization.

Observations of responses to heart surgery and to serial kidney biopsies yielded evidence of anxiety (Barnes, 1969; Mandleco, 1976). While limited detail of Barnes's study was reported, both behavioral observations and urine steroid levels reflected anxiety and stress among the 6- to 12-year-old youths (N = unreported). Mandleco's data, derived from interview, observation, and projective testing with 11 youths aged 5 to 13 years revealed evidence of denial, displacement, anxiety, and fear of the hospital experience. Altered postdischarge patterns in eating, sleeping, and play also were found. Parents reported that the children discussed the procedures, but not their feelings. Maintenance of control and limited feeling expression among schoolagers that would be predicted from developmental theory were evident in the Mandleco (1976) and Youssef (1981) data.

Content analysis of interview data from five 7- to 12-year-old hospitalized children with binocular bandages revealed restrictive verbal and nonverbal communication patterns and a focus on self (Riddle, 1972). More relaxed, meaningful communication and attention to others were evident when the bandages were removed and vision returned. No mental confusion or sensory and perceptual disturbances during the period of bandaging were evident. While the descriptive data from the Riddle (1972), Mandleco (1976), Neff (1978), and Youssef (1981) studies were gathered from small convenience samples, a particular strength of each investigation was the inclusion of specific behavioral data that illustrated the children's responses to health care procedures.

Responses of 44 children to pain associated with immunization were observed and then measured on two projective tests (Hester, 1979). Observed verbal, vocal, facial, and motor responses of those 4- to 8-year-old children correlated in varying degrees with one or both of the projective tests. While the study contributed information about assessment of children's responses to painful health care procedures, greater rigor in developing and testing of instrumentation would be needed before conclusions could be drawn about the quality of the measures.

Responses of 45 healthy young men aged 13 to 17 years to the potential of having their physical examination conducted by a woman reflected a moderate degree of concern in relation to body image, identity, independence, and relatedness (Mitchell, 1980). Age and an overall concern score were correlated negatively. Inclusion of instrument items, detailed descriptive data, and correlation matrices added greatly to the value of the report.

In summary, a limited number of instruments designed to measure youths' responses to chronic health problems, hospitalization, and health care procedures were developed and tested. Data regarding responses to chronic health problems such as amputation, scoliosis, hemophilia, cystic fibrosis, and cerebral palsy were generated. Patterns and themes of responses during hospitalization and health care procedures were evident.

THERAPEUTIC NURSING INTERVENTIONS WITH CHILDREN AND ADOLESCENTS

Therapeutic nursing interventions constituted the third major area of inquiry with schoolage children and adolescents. The interventions studied were directed toward health assessment; health education and health promotion; stress, distress, and anxiety alleviation; targeted social behavioral change; and physical health status alteration. Also included were a few studies that focused on practice settings in which nursing interventions were carried out.

Health Assessment

Nursing research related to health assessment included study of health problem appraisals (Tianen, 1962), body movement patterns (Downs & Fitzpatrick, 1976; Fitzpatrick & Donovan, 1979), body temperature

(Nicols, Kulvi, Life, & Christ, 1972), and vaginal organisms (Daus & Hafez, 1975). The process of health problem assessment and findings among 149 culturally deprived students ($N = 117$, grades 8, 9; $N = 32$ mentally handicapped classes) were described by Tianen (1962). Data from physical examinations, laboratory studies, vision and hearing screening, dental examination, and school records revealed health problems similar to those of the general youth population, but occurring to a greater degree. While comparative national data were not included, the pervasiveness of health problems was striking. Ninety-four percent of the students were judged to be in need of public health nursing services. This clearly written report was augmented by tabular presentation of data, but lacked any citations of related work.

Downs and Fitzpatrick (1976) developed an instrument to assess body position, gross motor activity, and intensity of motor activity. Initial reliability and validity estimates for the instrument were determined from testing with 14 children, aged 4 to 7 years. Additional reliability and validity testing was subsequently done with an adult population (Fitzpatrick & Donovan, 1979). Particular strengths of the investigation were (a) an explicit nursing context for the research, (b) a detailed description of the instrument development process, and (c) the yield of an instrument to measure body movement patterns within specified time periods in laboratory, field, and clinical settings.

Assessment of body temperature in febrile children was studied by Nichols et al. (1972). Data gathered from 50 children aged 7 to 13 years attending a hospital clinic revealed that traditional times of three to five minutes were insufficient for obtaining accurate oral temperatures. Optimum placement time was seven minutes for febrile children. Data from 40 children, aged 1 to 6, revealed that optimum placement for rectal temperature readings was four minutes. Significant differences in optimum placement by gender were noted for rectal, but not oral temperature readings. With the exception of information about specific statistical tests used, the research process was clearly articulated. Relevance for nursing practice was evident. A final strength of the study was that it was part of a program of research on measurement of body temperature in progress by the senior author and her colleagues.

Nursing assessment for the presence of *Candida albicans,* an organism responsible for the vaginal infection, *candidiasis,* was described by Daus and Hafez (1975). Although children and adolescents were included in the study, their data were not identified separately; thus examination of those data was impossible.

Research related to health assessment was extremely limited in quantity and diverse in content focus. In two of the studies, measurements of general health parameters were investigated (i.e., body temperature and body movement); in the other two, health problems and pathology were central to the research focus.

Health Education and Health Promotion

Areas of inquiry related to educative and health promotion nursing interventions with children and adolescents included self-care (Lewis et al., 1977; Pridham, 1971), health teaching about dental hygiene (Jeanes & Grant, 1976) and about nutrition (Rotatori, Parrish, & Freagon, 1979), and adolescent consent for health care (Jellinek, 1980). Lewis et al. and Pridham found that when nursing interventions designed to enhance youths' abilities to participate in their own health care were initiated, they responded with evidence of increased self-care competence. Children aged 5 to 12 years ($N = 309$) from a nongraded school responded to implementation of a child-initiated nursing services program by becoming involved in seeking health care and in the decision-making processes related to their health concerns (Lewis et al., 1977). Several demographic variables were significant predictors of utilization of the program. Use of multivariate analysis techniques strengthened the study.

In a descriptive case study, Pridham (1971) examined nursing interventions designed to instruct a 10-year-old girl with diabetes mellitus about increased responsibility for self-care. The intervention process of assessment of readiness, planning for removal of barriers to learning, and attending to and using child cues for readiness in learning were clearly described. This research provided a sound, scholarly, clinical case description built upon a theoretical and empirical base. Synthesis of nursing practice, theory, and research was enhanced by a clear, organized presentation.

The nursing intervention of health teaching yielded long- and short-term improvements in dental health (Jeanes & Grant, 1976) and short-term improvements in weight loss (Rotatori et al., 1979). An instructional intervention addressing toothbrushing technique, nutritional knowledge, and plaque control in 23 hospitalized youths, aged 4 to 13 years, resulted in improvements in all three areas during hospitalization. Sustained improvement postdischarge was found only in the brushing technique (Jeanes & Grant, 1976). A combination of parental instruction in nutrition and use of behavioral weight reduction techniques with six mildly and moderately retarded public school children resulted in an average weekly weight loss of .6 pounds (Rotatori et al., 1979). While the intervention used by the school nurse was clearly described, information was not reported about data collection and analysis. It was assumed that convenience samples were used in both studies.

Jellinek (1980) reported that health care providers and 50 youths in a general hospital adolescent clinic lacked knowledge of laws governing adolescents' rights to consent for health care. Limitations in reporting of the research process and the data made it difficult to draw specific conclusions.

With health promotion regularly identified as a major goal in nursing, it was encouraging to see studies in which the investigators addressed educative and health promotion interventions. Although limited, data were generated on the effectiveness of nursing interventions designed to enhance children's self-care competence, dental hygiene, and nutritional or weight status. The need for development of educative nursing interventions related to minors' consent for health care also was suggested by the research.

Stress, Distress, and Anxiety Alleviation

Nursing interventions involving preparation of children for health care experiences were effective in reducing or alleviating stress, distress, and anxiety. Six to 11-year-old children prepared for orthopedic cast removal by hearing a taped message describing physical sensations associated with the procedure displayed less distress than did children who received no experimental information (Johnson, Kirchhoff, & Endress, 1975, 1976). Eighty-four children were assigned randomly to three information groups: taped sensation information, taped procedural information, and no taped information. Only the sensation information significantly reduced distress. Strengths of the study were clear articulation of the conceptualization that congruency between expected and experienced sensations would reduce distress, rigorous attention to research procedures, and careful presentation of multivariate analysis. The research of Johnson and her colleagues was also one of the few examples in nursing of the careful building of a research program designed to test a hypothesis in multiple situations.

Children who received the experimental intervention of systematic psychologic preparation and continued supportive nursing care demonstrated less upset behavior and more cooperation in the hospital and fewer posthospital adjustment problems than did children who did not receive the experimental intervention (McGrath, 1979; Wolfer & Visintainer, 1975). The Wolfer and Visintainer experimental study of 80 hospitalized youths aged 3 to 14 years was methodologically sound, carefully conceptualized, and relevant to practice. The McGrath study of 44 3- to 12-year-old youths, was built carefully upon the Wolfer and Visintainer research but used group rather than individual preparation and supportive care during hospitalization. Analysis and results of the McGrath study were less clearly reported than were other aspects of the research.

Naylor, Kan, and Coates (1982) found that 3- to 6-year-old children who experienced vicarious preparation for cardiac catheterization demonstrated less overt regressive, aggressive, and anxiety behaviors at home following the procedure and less crying, calling for mother, complaints of pain, and motor activity during the procedure than did those children who received routine preparation ($N = 30$). Vicarious preparation included use of behavioral rehearsal, manuals, and coloring books by which individual coping strategies could be identified and practiced. While limited data about this experimental study were available, there was evidence that the nursing intervention was effective in reducing distress.

Hedberg and Schlong (1973) demonstrated that an instructional intervention focused on expected role behaviors (i.e., that children were to remain on their feet at all times and not faint or fuss) was effective in reducing fainting and other disruptive behavior during mass inoculation. None of the 2,338 students receiving the experimental instructions fainted or displayed disruptive behavior during the procedure; 18 of the 1,978 students in the control group receiving neutral instructions either fainted or displayed disruptive behavior. Although some details of data collection were omitted and no related work was cited, the strength of the study lay in the testing of a specific nursing intervention with a very large sample. Inclusion of the actual text of the preparatory instruction message was viewed as potentially useful for future nursing research and practice.

A nursing intervention involving a carefully planned teaching-learning experience about hospitalization was effective in changing drawings by 30 6-to 12-year old children from unrealistic, fearful representations to realistic, confident depictions of what it would be like to be in the hospital (Allen, 1978). The intervention included a slide presentation, discussion, and play related to hospital experiences and sensations. Although limited detail regarding the analysis was reported, the postintervention drawings appeared to reflect a reduction in confusion, fearfulness, and/or ignorance associated with hospitalization.

Several other studies of interventions involving preparation for hospital experiences yielded mixed and unclear results (Crocker, 1980; Meng, 1980; Williams, 1980). Williams (1980) compared the effectiveness of story, story and play, and neither story nor play in reducing postoperative distress in 7- to 12-year-old Filipino children. Crocker (1980) tested a film puppet show, discussion, and free play intervention with 4- to 10-year-old children. Meng's (1980) preadmission intervention of a videotaped puppet show and discussion designed to reduce anxiety was tested with 4- to 10-year-old children. Difficulties encountered during the course of the Williams study and limitations in presentation of Crocker's and Meng's research made interpretation of the findings difficult.

In a study by Menke (1981), no relationship was found between preparation for hospital and stimuli perceived as stressful by 50 6- to 12-year-old children. However, the research yielded valuable descriptive data about children's perceptions of stressful stimuli. The study was built carefully upon previous research; attention to reliability and validity was evident in the development of the measurement process; and an instrument for evaluating potentially stressful stimuli was developed for use in future research and practice.

In several nursing intervention studies, investigators described use of play to reduce stress or anxiety associated with hospital experiences (Clatworthy, 1981; Lockwood, 1970; Oestreich, 1969). Oestreich (1969) used play with hospital equipment and family figures before and after cardiac catheterization for six children aged 6 to 17 years. Lockwood (1970) tested the effect of situational doll play on preoperative stress levels of 20 4- to 6-year-old children. Clatworthy (1981) examined the effect of daily therapeutic play experiences on anxiety in 114 children aged 5 to 12 years. Oestreich's report contained a clear description of the play experience, but only data on one of the six children were reported. Lockwood found that doll play did not affect preoperative stress. Use of randomization and discussion of play as a communication tool with children were strengths of Lockwood's work; the lack of data to support the author's conclusions was a limitation. Clatworthy found that play was a deterrent to increase in anxiety among hospitalized youth. Anxiety of children receiving play was essentially the same at admission and discharge; anxiety of children not receiving play was higher at discharge than at admission (alpha level = .01). This experimental study was more carefully designed and reported than were the earlier works.

Two intervention studies involving parents in the care of hospitalized children were reported (Mahaffy, 1965; White & Wear, 1980). In the Mahaffy research (1965), an experimental nursing intervention comprised of parental involvement and support led to significantly less distress among 43 2- to 10-year-old hospitalized children than did routine care in which parent interaction was limited. Methodological, theoretical, and practice aspects were sound and well reported. In the White and Wear (1980) study, interventions involving the use of stories tape recorded for the child by a parent absent at bedtime and/or nightly phone calls to the parent by a nurse were studied in relation to 3- to 8-year-old children's going to sleep behaviors (N = unreported). Analysis was incomplete at the time of reporting. Promising technology for data recordings was noted, but unfortunately, in the interest of brevity of reporting, clarity of both technology and content was sacrificed.

Collectively the nursing studies related to stress, distress, and anxiety reduction yielded considerable data, especially with respect to the effectiveness of various approaches to preparation for hospital experiences. A wide variety of interventions was tested with the youths and with their parents. Patterns of effective strategies for stress, distress, and anxiety reduction were evident; differentiations among them were not clearly refined.

Targeted Social Behavioral Change

Investigators studying nursing interventions directed toward targeted social behavioral change in children and adolescents focused on reduction of hyperactive behavior (Pratt & Fischer, 1975), facilitation and measurement of verbal and nonverbal social interaction behaviors (Balthazar, English, & Sindberg, 1971; Hinds, 1980; Spurgeon, 1967), and imitation as a means of social learning (Harbin, Sklar, & Trautman, 1969). An operant reinforcement (behavior modification) intervention program was studied and found effective in reducing hyperactive behavior in a 9-year-old in a group setting on an inpatient psychiatric unit (Pratt & Fischer, 1975). An experimental nursing program combining operant reinforcement and nurturant, supportive, personalized interventions resulted in improvement in three areas of social behavior among 16 residents of a residential center for persons with mental retardation (Balthazar et al., 1971). Improvements were in the areas of unskilled verbalization, failure to respond to contact by others, and nonverbal communication.

Hinds (1980) found that social interaction behaviors during group play therapy were significantly higher for 10 low-income Mexican-American boys, aged 8 to 10 years, during periods when music was added than during periods without music. The behavioral changes associated with music were increases in verbalization, proximity with peers and therapists, and involvement with toy exchanges. Inconsistencies in portions of the analysis presentation necessitated caution in drawing conclusions, but there was evidence that in selected situations, music was a promising nursing intervention for enhancing social interaction skills. In the Spurgeon (1967) research, results of nursing intervention designed to enhance social interaction patterns of three 9- and 10-year-old autistic children were unclear, but the description of the process and problems associated with instrument development was valuable. Discussion of observation and content analysis issues was thoughtfully done.

Harbin et al. (1969) found that 20 emotionally disturbed youths learned by imitation in a manner similar to 20 clinically normal youths. The conceptual basis for this laboratory study was modeling and behavioral theory. The number of trials to imitation of a model's game behavior was compared across groups. The potential of imitation for learning appropriate social behaviors from nursing models was addressed. The Harbin research and the other nursing intervention studies directed toward social behavioral change yielded data on use of behavioral techniques separately and in combination with supportive, nurturant care; use of music to augment group play therapy; instrumentation for measuring nonverbal autistic behavior; and imitative learning.

Physical Health Status Alteration

In two nursing studies, investigators examined interventions directed toward alteration of specific aspects of physical health status in children and adolescents. Clément, Jankowski, and Beaudry (1979) found physical work capacity and maximal oxygen consumption increased in three youths with cystic fibrosis, aged 6 to 15 years, who completed a program of prone immersion exercise. The exercise intervention consisted of tethered swimming with fin and kickboard three times weekly for 26 weeks. Strengths of this pilot study were careful description of the research process, the investigator's use of related research with adults, and the yield of a potential alternative for standard chest therapy with youths with cystic fibrosis.

In a double blind investigation, Shields, Hovey, and Fuller (1980) found that neither meperidine nor physostigmine, two medications regularly prescribed for alleviation of emergent excitement, was more effective than a sodium chloride placebo. The study sample was comprised of 59 healthy children aged 2 to 13 years recovering from posttonsillectomy anesthesia. Presentation was directed toward the practitioner but adequately addressed research aspects. A study synopsis figure that contained the key points of the research was a valuable addition to the report. These two studies related to physical health status provided data about effectiveness of nursing interventions and as such raised questions about and suggested alternatives to current nursing practices.

Nursing Practice in Home, Camp, and School Settings

In the final cluster of nursing studies reviewed, the investigators addressed structure and process of nursing practice in home, camp, and school settings. The development of home care programs for the dying child and nurses' attitudes toward those programs were studied by Martinson, Palta, and Rude (1978) and by Moldow and Martinson (1980). Details of data collection and analysis were limited. The contribution of the studies lay primarily in their part in an ongoing program of research, service, and education related to care of children and families. Godbout and Hurwitz (1960) studied utilization of camp nursing services. Reasons for visits obtained from camp records were described. However, no detail of the research process was included.

Several nursing investigators addressed school health issues. Ehling (1955) examined factors associated with adoption and application of school health records. Data collection approaches and conclusions about the record system were clearly described, but the lack of a description of analysis limited the value of this report. In their study of characteristics of school nurses, Cauffman, Casady, Randall, Warburton, and Schultz (1969) found that socioeconomic background, number of offspring, and professional preparation of the nurses were associated with whether or not children received follow-up care for health problems. In a study conceptualized within a nursing systems theory framework, Stamler and Palmer (1971) found dependency characteristics among children who made repeated visits to the school nurse were significantly greater than among children who did not make repeated visits. Although not sophisticated, the analyses for these two studies were adequate. Generally, these early studies of nurse and client characteristics and utilization of nursing services in camp and school settings provided limited but potentially relevant data which may direct future research and practice.

SUMMARY, RESEARCH DIRECTIONS

The accumulated knowledge base to date for nursing practice with school-age children and adolescents was found to be tenuous and fragmented. Approximately one hundred nursing studies were identified and reviewed. Among those studies were examples of research in which conceptual, methodological, and practice related issues were addressed in a thorough, scholarly manner. However, those examples were extremely few in number. Only a small number of reports reflected any explicit attention to the conceptual or theoretical basis of study. Quality of reported research methods was often very limited; analysis techniques frequently were not cited. Relevance of the studies to nursing practice was often implicit, but on many occasions the word nursing did not even appear. Collectively the studies reflected a distressing lack of attention to scholarly study of related empirical and theoretical works.

There are many concepts relevant or essential to nursing's knowledge base for practice about which there are beginning data or about which there is need to generate data. The fragmented approach to nursing research is of especial concern. Barnard and Neal (1977) expressed a similar concern based on their review of maternal-child nursing research. If an adequate knowledge base for nursing practice is to be generated, it is imperative that research be pursued in a scholarly manner that takes into account not only work from other disciplines, but also carefully studies and builds upon the work of the discipline of nursing. Programs of research centered around concepts central to the discipline must be mounted if nursing is to achieve the desired knowledge base for practice.

It is of less concern at this stage *which* conceptual schema is used than it is that *some* conceptual schema are used in nursing investigations. It is because of that concern that major attention in this review was given to the development of a conceptual clustering within which to view the research to date. The identification of the three major areas of inquiry (i.e., [1] child and adolescent perceptions of and [2] responses to self, life events, and environment; and nursing interventions directed toward particular outcomes) also provides one pattern of conceptual organization that can be used for future development of a scientific knowledge base for nursing practice with youths and their families.

Based on this conceptual organization, it is clear that nursing's accumulated knowledge to date includes data about youths' knowledge and perceptions of themselves in terms of health and their knowledge and perceptions about illness, death, and locus of control. Data about child and adolescent responses to general life change events, fear events, violence, moving, disability in a parent, chronic health problems, hospitalization, and health care procedures also are available. Patterns of response to procedures and hospitalization are emerging; more careful study will be required to explicate and test those patterns. Knowledge about effectiveness of nursing interventions is uneven. Knowledge about strategies for stress, distress, and anxiety reduction is strongest; knowledge of health assessment and health promotion is least well developed.

There was marked development in the quality of research methods reflected in nursing studies with children and adolescents over the last 30 years. The recent research was more carefully designed and more adequately reported than that of earlier years. While strengths of the studies were identified and growth was apparent, collectively the limitations were considerable. Frequently the population from which the sample was drawn and the sampling plan were unclear or unspecified. Reliability and validity of instruments were often questionable, not determined, or not reported. Data collection procedures often were addressed inadequately. Least clear of all were the selection, use, and understanding of data analysis techniques; this lack compromised the presentation of the results.

In future nursing research related to schoolage children and adolescents, both conceptual and methodological aspects need to be addressed. The current data base needs to be studied and respected in terms of both strengths and limitations. With nursing's goal of maintenance and promotion of health, increased attention must be placed on studying the knowledge, attitude, and skill resources children and adolescents have available for health promotion. While responses to illness have been studied to a degree, general health practices and health status of youth have been virtually unexplored. There is need for examination of nursing interventions designed to enhance the health resources, health practices, and health status of youth. The knowledge base for nursing practice with children and adolescents will become increasingly sound if there is continued research in areas in which knowledge is being accumulated and if increased effort is exerted in areas such as health promotion. The quality of the future knowledge base also will be heavily dependent upon the thoroughness and rigor of the development, implementation, and reporting of the research efforts in nursing.

REFERENCES

Allen, J. M. Influencing school-age children's concept of hospitalization. *Pediatric Nursing*, 1978, *4*(6), 26–28.

Astin, E. W. Self reported fears of hospitalized and non-hospitalized children aged ten to twelve. *Maternal-Child Nursing Journal*, 1977, *6*, 17–24.

Balthazar, E. E., English, G. E., & Sindberg, R. M. Behavior changes in mentally retarded children following the initiation of an experimental nursing program. *Nursing Research*, 1971, *20*, 69–74.

Barnard, K. E., & Neal, M. V. Maternal-child nursing research: Review of the past and present strategies for the future. *Nursing Research*, 1977, *26*, 193–200.

Barnes, C. M. Working with parents of children undergoing heart surgery. *Nursing Clinics of North America*, 1969, *4*(1), 11–18.

Barnes, C. M. Levels of consciousness indicated by responses of children to pneumonia in the intensive care unit. *Maternal-Child Nursing Journal*, 1975, *4*, 215–290. (Monograph)

Beard, M. T. Interpersonal trust, life events and coping in an ethnic adolescent population. *Journal of Psychiatric Nursing and Mental Health Services*, 1980, *18*(11), 12–20.

Benoliel, J. Q. The developing diabetic identity: A study of family influence. In M. V. Batey (Ed.), *Communicating nursing research* (Vol. 3). Boulder, Colo.: Western Interstate Commission for Higher Education, 1970.

Brodie, B. Views of healthy children toward illness. *American Journal of Public Health*, 1974, *64*, 1156–1159.

Burgess, A. W., & Holmstrom, L. L. Crisis and counseling requests of rape victims. *Nursing Research*, 1974, *23*, 196–202.

Cauffman, J. G., Casady, L. L., Randall, H. B., Warburton, E. A., & Schultz, C. S. The nurse and health care of school children, *Nursing Research*, 1969, *18*, 412–417.

Clatworthy, S. Therapeutic play: Effects on hospitalized children. *Journal of the Association for the Care of Children's Health*, 1981, *9*, 108–113.

Clément, M., Jankowski, L. W., & Beaudry, P. H. Prone immersion physical exercise therapy in three children with cystic fibrosis: A pilot study. *Nursing Research*, 1979, *28*, 325–329.

Craft, M. Preferences of hopitalized adolescents for information providers. *Nursing Research*, 1981, *30*, 205–211.

Crocker, E. Preparation for elective surgery: Does it make a difference? *Journal of the Association for the Care of Children's Health*, 1980, *9*, 3–11.

Daubenmire, M. J., Pierce, L. M., & Weaver, B. R. Adolescence in the hospital. *Nursing Outlook*, 1960, *8*, 502–504.

Daus, A. D., & Hafez, E. S. E. Candida albicans in women. *Nursing Research*, 1975, *24*, 431–433.

Denyes, M. J. Measurement of self-care agency in adolescents. *Nursing Research*, 1982, *31*, 63. (Abstract)

Downs, F. S., & Fitzpatrick, J. J. Preliminary investigation of the reliability and validity of a tool for the assessment of body position and motor activity. *Nursing Research*, 1976, *25*, 404–408.

Eggland, E. T. Locus of control and children with cerebral palsy. *Nursing Research*, 1973, *22*, 329–333.

Ehling, C. L. School health records in health counseling of children and parents. *Nursing Research*, 1955, *4*, 90–91.

Fitzpatrick, J. J., & Donovan, M. J. A follow-up study of the reliability and validity of the Motor Activity Rating Scale. *Nursing Research*, 1979, *28*, 179–181.

Garlinghouse, J., & Sharp, L. J. The hemophilic child's self-concept and family stress in relation to bleeding episodes. *Nursing Research*, 1968, *17*, 32–37.

Godbout, R. A., & Hurwitz, I. The role of the infirmary in a therapeutic camp for boys. *Nursing Research*, 1960, *9*, 23–31.

Hagemann, V. Night sleep of children in a hospital. Part I: Sleep duration. *Maternal-Child Nursing Journal*, 1981, *10*, 1–13. (a)

Hagemann, V. Night sleep of children in a hospital. Part II: Sleep disruption. *Maternal-Child Nursing Journal*, 1981, *10*, 127–142. (b)

Harbin, A. L., Sklar, C. L., & Trautman, E. M. A study of imitative learning in emotionally disturbed and normal children. *Nursing Research*, 1969, *18*, 160–164.

Hedberg, A. G., & Schlong, A. Eliminating fainting by school children during mass inoculation clinics. *Nursing Research*, 1973, *22*, 352–353.

Hester, N. K. O. The preoperational child's reaction to immunization. *Nursing Research*, 1979, *28*, 250–255.

Hinds, P. S. Music: A milieu factor with implications for the nurse-therapist. *Journal of Psychiatric Nursing and Mental Health Services*, 1980, *18*(6), 28–33.

Holaday, B. J. Achievement behavior in chronically ill children. *Nursing Research*, 1974, *23*, 25–30.

Jeanes, K. R., & Grant, J. R. Children's retention of dental hygiene instruction. *Nursing Research*, 1976, *25*, 452–454.

Jellinek, B. J. Adolescents' knowledge of consent laws in a Massachusetts community. *Pediatric Nursing*, 1980, *6*(2), 21–23.

Johnson, J. E., Kirchhoff, K. T., & Endress, M. P. Altering children's distress behavior during orthopedic cast removal. *Nursing Research*, 1975, *24*, 404–410.

Johnson, J. E., Kirchhoff, K. T., & Endress, M. P. Easing children's fright during health care procedures. *MCN, American Journal of Maternal Child Nursing*, 1976, *1*, 206–210.

Kueffner, M. Passage through hospitalization of severely burned, isolated school-age children. In M. V. Batey (Ed.), *Communicating nursing research* (Vol. 7). Boulder, Colo.: Western Interstate Commission for Higher Education, 1975.

Lewis, C. E., Lewis, M. A., Lorimer, A., & Palmer, B. B. Child-initiated care: The use of school nursing services by children in an "adult-free" system. *Pediatrics*, 1977, *60*, 499–507.

Lockwood, N. L. The effect of situational doll play upon the preoperative stress reactions of hospitalized children. In American Nurses' Association, *ANA clinical sessions*. New York: Appleton-Century-Crofts, 1970.

Mahaffy, P. R. The effects of hospitalization on children admitted for tonsillectomy and adenoidectomy. *Nursing Research*, 1965, *14*, 12–19.

Mandleco, B. Nursing assessment of children undergoing kidney biopsy. *Maternal-Child Nursing Journal*, 1976, *5*, 151–166.

Martinson, I. M., Palta, M., & Rude, N. V. Death and dying: Selected attitudes of Minnesota's registered nurses. *Nursing Research*, 1978, *27*, 226–229.

McGrath, M. M. Group preparation of pediatric surgical patients. *Image*, 1979, *11*, 52–62.

Mendez, L. K., Yeaworth, R. C., York, J. A., & Goodwin, T. Factors influencing adolescents' perceptions of life change events. *Nursing Research*, 1980, *29*, 384–388.

Meng, A. L. Parents' and children's reactions toward impending hospitalization for surgery. *Maternal-Child Nursing Journal*, 1980, *9*, 83–98.

Menke, E. M. School-aged children's perception of stress in the hospital. *Journal of the Association for the Care of Children's Health*, 1981, *9*, 80–86.

Miller, S. Children's fears: A review of the literature with implications for nursing research and practice. *Nursing Research*, 1979, *28*, 217–223.

Mitchell, J. R. Male adolescents' concern about a physical examination conducted by a female. *Nursing Research*, 1980, *29*, 165–169.

Moldow, D. G., & Martinson, I. M. From research to reality—Home care for the dying child. *MCN, American Journal of Maternal Child Nursing*, 1980, *5*, 159–162, 166.

Nathan, S. W. Body image of scoliotic female adolescents before and after surgery. *Maternal-Child Nursing Journal*, 1977, *6*, 139–149.

Naylor, D., Kan, J. S., & Coates, T. J. Reducing stress in pediatric cardiac catheterization. *Nursing Research*, 1982, *31*, 127.

Neff, E. J. A. Orienting, resistive and adaptive responses of children undergoing hemodialysis for kidney failure. *Maternal-Child Nursing Journal*, 1978, *7*, 195–254. (Monograph)

Nichols, G. A., Kulvi, R. L., Life, H. R., & Christ, N. M. Measuring oral and rectal temperatures of febrile children. *Nursing Research*, 1972, *21*, 261–264.

Oestreich, P. Children's reactions to cardiac catheterization. *Nursing Clinics of North America*, 1969, *4*(1), 3–10.

Olgas, M. The relationship between parents' health status and body image of their children. *Nursing Research*, 1974, *23*, 319–324.

Porter, C. S. Grade school children's perceptions of their internal body parts. *Nursing Research*, 1974, *23*, 384–391.

Pratt, S. J., & Fischer, J. Behavior modification: Changing hyperactive behavior in a children's group. *Perspectives in Psychiatric Care*, 1975, *13*, 37–42.

Pridham, K. F. Instruction of a school-age child with chronic illness for increased responsibility in self-care, using diabetes mellitus as an example. *International Journal of Nursing Studies*, 1971, *8*, 237–246.

Quiggin, V. Children's knowledge of their internal body parts. *Nursing Times*, 1977, *73*, 1146–1151.

Riddle, I. I. Communicative behaviors of hospitalized school age children with binocular bandages. *Maternal-Child Nursing Journal*, 1972, *1*, 291–354. (Monograph)

Riffee, D. M. Self-esteem changes in hospitalized school-age children. *Nursing Research*, 1981, *30*, 94–97.

Ritchie, J. A. Adjustive and affective responses of school-aged children to a leg amputation. *Nursing Papers*, 1977, *9*(3), 103–107. (Abstract) (a)

Ritchie, J. Children's adjustive and affective responses in the process of reformulating a body image following limb amputation. *Maternal-Child Nursing Journal*, 1977, *6*, 25–34. (b)

Ritchie, J. A. Nursing the child undergoing limb amputation. *MCN, American Journal of Maternal Child Nursing*, 1980, *5*, 114–120.

Rodgers, B., Ferholt, J., & Cooper, C. L. A screening tool to detect psychosocial adjustment of children with cystic fibrosis. *Nursing Research*, 1974, *23*, 420–426.

Rotatori, A. F., Parrish, P., & Freagon, S. Weight loss in retarded children—A pilot study. *Journal of Psychiatric Nursing and Mental Health Services*, 1979, *17*(10), 33–34.

Savedra, M., & Tesler, M. Coping strategies of hospitalized school-age children. *Western Journal of Nursing Research*, 1981, *3*, 371–384.

Shields, J. R., Hovey, J. K., & Fuller, S. S. A comparison of physostigmine and meperidine in treating emergence excitement. *MCN, American Journal of Maternal Child Nursing*, 1980, *5*, 170–175.

Spurgeon, R. K. Some problems in measuring nonverbal behavior of autistic children. *Nursing Research*, 1967, *16*, 212–218.

Stamler, C., & Palmer, J. O. Dependency and repetitive visits to the nurse's office in elementary school children. *Nursing Research*, 1971, *20*, 254–255.

Stoll, C. Responses of three girls to burn injuries and hospitalization. *Nursing Clinics of North America*, 1969, *4*(1), 77–87.

Swain, H. L. Childhood views of death. *Death Education*, 1979, *2*, 341–358.

Tesler, M., & Savedra, M. Coping with hospitalization: A study of school-age children. *Pediatric Nursing*, 1981, *7*(2), 35–38.

Tianen, D. A. Analytic study of the physical findings of the health appraisals of culturally deprived children. *Nursing Research*, 1962, *11*, 231–233.

Van Dongen, C. J. Relationships between attitudes toward family change of residence and children's postmove adjustment. *Issues in Mental Health Nursing*, 1981, *3*, 51–62.

Weiss, H. A ward adjustment and behavior rating schedule for children and adolescents in residential psychiatric settings. *Nursing Research*, 1969, *18*, 357–363.

Westra, B., & Martin, H. P. Children of battered women. *Maternal-Child Nursing Journal*, 1981, *10*, 41–54.

White, M. A., & Wear, E. Parent-child separation: An observational methodology. *Western Journal of Nursing Research*, 1980, *2*, 759–760.

Williams, P. D. A comparison of Philippine and American children's concepts of body organs and illness in relation to five variables. *International Journal of Nursing Studies*, 1978, *15*, 193–202.

Williams, P. D. Preparation of school-age children for surgery: A program in

preventive pediatrics—Philippines. *International Journal of Nursing Studies*, 1980, *17*, 107–119.
Wolfer, J. A., & Visintainer, M. A. Pediatric surgical patients' and parents' stress responses and adjustment. *Nursing Research*, 1975, *24*, 244–255.
Yanni, M. I. Perception of parents' behavior and children's general fearfulness. *Nursing Research*, 1982, *31*, 79–82.
Yeaworth, R. C., York, J. A., Hussey, M. A., Ingle, E., & Goodwin, T. The development of an adolescent life change event scale. *Adolescence*, 1980, *15*, 91–97.
Youssef, M. M. S. Self-control behaviors of school-age children who are hospitalized for cardiac diagnostic procedures. *Maternal-Child Nursing Journal*, 1981, *10*, 219–284. (Monograph)

CHAPTER 3

Adulthood: A Promising Focus for Future Research

JOANNE SABOL STEVENSON
SCHOOL OF NURSING
OHIO STATE UNIVERSITY

CONTENTS

Adulthood is an elusive topic for critical research review. While much nursing research is focused upon people 18 to 70 years old, little of it actually is about adults as adults. Nursing has not to date "discovered" the enormous potential of health-related research and theory building about adults as growing, maturing human beings. Research on child development has a rich tradition in nursing, and in recent years efforts have been made to study adolescence and aging as developmental stages. But no discernible research attention has been devoted to the maturational aspects of adulthood.

While the nursing profession espouses a developmental approach, it has been content to borrow theories from other disciplines, primarily

The author wishes to thank Louise Anderson, Barbara Smith, and Dr. Mary Irene Moffitt for their assistance with technical aspects of this project.

developmental psychology. Nursing would benefit from having a knowledge base about adult development under conditions of health promotion, ill health, and crisis conditions. Hence, it would behoove nurse researchers to become involved in developmentally oriented research.

Since there was minimal research to review and critique, the author chose to search the literature where developmentally oriented research could have been but was not present. Decision rules governing the selection of literature included the following: (a) age, life stage, or developmentally linked crisis was a component of the phenomena under study, although the investigator may not have attended to this component; (b) illness-oriented research was included if the illness experience had the potential to impact on progress in adult development, whether or not this impact was given attention by the investigator; and (c) research that actually used developmental concepts or developmental issues as theoretical underpinnings of the study.

Since the approach taken in this chapter was to critique what could have been but was not present in the literature, the theoretical frameworks and major variables were the primary foci for scrutiny. Full methodological critiques of the studies were not included here. It is envisioned that the major contribution of this chapter will be a developmentally oriented model for future research on adulthood in nursing. To this end a schematic model is presented for consideration by the nursing research community.

NURSING'S INTEREST IN ADULTHOOD

Substantive information about biological and psychosocial growth and development during the ages and stages of adult life has been provided in chapters in nursing textbooks that cover the whole life span; this trend began in the early 1970s. Examples published recently are: Bornstein, 1980; Draheim and Ashburn, 1980; Ebersole and Hess, 1981; and Mourad, 1980. Only one entire nursing textbook (Stevenson, 1977) has been devoted to growth and development during adulthood. Adulthood as a life stage is also included in chapters of textbooks on other topics, such as crisis and family therapy (Aguilera, Messick, & Farrell, 1970; Hall, 1974; Williams, 1974), and in clinical journals (Dennis, 1981; Diekelmann, 1975, 1976; Hargreaves, 1975). The implication of this attention to stages of adulthood is that human development theories comprise a necessary learning experience for nursing students and hence have implications for nursing practice. Unfortunately, except for vignettes of illustrative single cases, the research covered in these writings is drawn from other fields; authors have not included original research from nursing sources. A review of this literature did not reveal narrative or bibliographic references to nursing studies of adult developmental issues. A glaring shortcoming of all the nursing textbooks reviewed was the absence of implications of nursing practice based on the developmental theories. The reason is self evident: without nursing oriented research and prescriptive theory emanating from such research (and vice versa) there is a paucity of valid recommendations for practice (Donaldson & Crowley, 1978). An academic discipline (i.e., developmental psychology) has only to produce descriptive theories, for there is no need to attend to applicability. A professional discipline (i.e., nursing) must go further and produce and test prescriptive theories. Otherwise, there is a gap between theory and practice, as there now is in the adult development literature in nursing.

Adult clients comprise a significant percentage of nursing's consumer population. It is incumbent upon nurses to develop knowledge about the normal life processes of this age group and to incorporate knowledge about normal adult development in studies about a variety of life experiences. Nurse researchers frequently measure phenomena such as parent bonding behavior, health behavior, locus of control, or impact of life change events. But what do these researchers incorporate in their theoretical frameworks about human maturation and its effect on the phenomena under study? The review of the nursing research literature that forms the basis of this chapter showed a poor grasp of fundamental knowledge about adult development and maturational change.

SIGNIFICANT ISSUES FOR THE MIDDLE YEARS

Four major areas of experience comprise the adult's life space: (a) family life, including the marital relationship and child-rearing functions; (b) work and leisure; (c) social participation and community responsibility; and (d) development of personal maturity, including physical aging of the body (Stevenson, 1977). Major developmental objectives have been delineated for the stages of adult life. Adult stages can be useful indirectly as contextual anchors for research on a myriad of adult phenomena. Adult life stages also can serve as points of departure for research questions directly targeted to build knowledge about developmental aspects of adulthood.

The stages of adult life and the major developmental objective of each stage are: (a) during young adulthood (18 to 30 years of age approximately), the major objective is to achieve relative independence from parental figures and a sense of responsibility (emotional, socioeconomic, and cultural) for one's own life; (b) during the core middle years (30 to 50 years of age approximately), the major objective is to assume responsibility for growth and development of self and of organizational enterprises, and a second objective is to provide help to younger and older generations; (c) during the new middle years (50 to 70 years of age approximately), the major objective is to assume primary responsibility for the continued survival and enhancement of the culture and larger social systems of mankind; and (d) during late adulthood (70 plus years of age), the major objective is to assume responsibility for sharing the wisdom of age, reviewing life, and putting affairs in order (Stevenson, 1977).

In the following sections, the author reviews nursing research in areas that correspond to the significant components of adult life. In each topic area an attempt was made to show how adult developmental theory could have provided a contextual underpinning to the studies, thus improving their potential meaningfulness for nursing.

PARENTING AS A MATURATIONAL FORCE

Parent-child (maternal-child) research is an area where investigators have ignored the human developmental aspect of the adult subjects. Studies found in this literature did not give evidence of an appropriate grounding in the knowledge base of the parents' (mothers') developmental stages and of the multiple and conflicting developmental tasks facing young adults. One study on adolescent pregnancy contained evidence of the investigator's sensitivity to the developmental age/stage of the pregnant teen (Thomas, 1979). But attention to development was absent in studies of adult pregnant subjects; these studies did not include focus on how the pregnancy influenced the mothers' development.

Earlier in its history, the maternal-child literature focused on the child as a primary and the mother as a secondary subject, of interest only in terms of her contribution to the child's welfare. Since the advent of the women's movement, the father has been acknowledged as a parent, but again primarily as a secondary subject in deference to the child.

Research reviewed on parent-child relationships and the parenting role was limited to titles that implied a focus on one or both parents. Several studies concerned with parental perception of personal competence (Bowen & Miller, 1980; Cronenwett & Newmark, 1974; Gruis, 1977; Kunst-Wilson & Cronenwett, 1981; Larsen, 1966; May, 1980; McCaffery & Johnson, 1967; Reiber, 1976; Rubin, 1967a, 1967b; Smith, 1965/1967; Willmuth, Weaver, & Borenstein, 1978) were reviewed. While the data collected targeted the parent-child relationship, the authors were concerned with the quality of the relationship from the perspective of the child's welfare. Hence, the parent as an adult was not truly a focus of attention.

One may argue that it is not the responsibility of parent-child researchers to concern themselves with the adult development of parents. No doubt that is a valid argument, but adult development should be the concern of someone in nursing, since parents equally are clients with the offspring. The logical solution would be collaborative research (or at least consultation) between the child health experts and experts in adult development. Research on parents as maturing human beings would provide valuable insights for the parent-child health arena. The child cannot be studied as a holistic being if researchers strip the parent of humanity by studying one role in isolation.

The critical review of research on father participation in child care by Cronenwett (1982) dealt tangentially with the issue of the potential benefits of active fathering as a maturing force for the father. It was one of the few articles to contain even indirect comments about parent maturation. The child-oriented focus on parents also was evident in the review of studies concerned with the stepparent-child relationship (Palermo, 1980; Stern, 1982) and with studies on single parenting (Hanson, 1981; Norbeck & Sheiner, 1982).

Mercer (1981), in a comprehensive review of the maternal role research literature, reported that of all the factors found to impact on the maternal role, "age is supported consistently as accounting for significant variance in mothering behaviors," (Mercer, 1981, p. 76). The problem here is that age has always been studied as a demographic variable; hence, it has had no interpretive meaning. But if age as developmental stage were to become a variable of interest, insightful findings might be derived from indepth studies of differences in maternal role behavior based on age/stage of adult development.

Studies of parental coping with acutely, chronically, and terminally ill children (Kessler, 1969; Merrow & Johnson, 1968; Nikolaisen & Williams, 1980; Skipper, Leonard, & Rhymes, 1968) dealt with disruptions in the household and impact of the illness on spouse-spouse and parent-sibling relationships. This attention to matters of adult life was descriptive only. There were no attempts made to fit the findings into a conceptual framework. Hence, the meaning of the findings remains obscure. No studies were found in nursing that focused on the parent as an adult fulfilling developmental tasks through the medium of procreation, parenting, or coping with the stress of childhood illness. The reports of Martinson (1979) and Martinson and Jorgens (1976) describing parents' caring for dying children contain spontaneous quotes from parents about their own growth during and after the terminal illness experience. These quotations were not analyzed in relation to theory about situational crises as maturing forces, but they are suggestive of areas for future research.

FAMILIAZATION AS A MATURATIONAL FORCE

Familiazation refers to the development of long-term, intimate relationships, whether the adult heads of family are engaged in traditional marital relationships, long-term cohabitation relationships of the common law or homosexual type, or have a single adult head (Stevenson, 1977). Variation currently is prevalent in the United States, but the same basic rules of family life prevail regardless of the form or style the family takes. Further, the familiazation either enhances or depresses the maturational progress of the adult members of the family (just as it does the child members); family life is not a neutral experience.

Duvall (1967), in her child-oriented conception of family life, defined stages of family development through the ages of the children. Stevenson (1977) argued that this approach was not useful for the study of adult development and designated stages of family life in terms of the longevity of family life-in-process (familiazation). The adult-oriented stages are: Stage I, the Emerging family—first 7 to 10 years of cohabitation; Stage II, the Crystallizing family—10 to 25 years of cohabitation; Stage III, the Integrating family—25 to 40 years of cohabitation; and Stage IV, the Actualizing family—40 to 60+ years of cohabitation. This manner of viewing family development lends itself to the reciprocal study of the growth and maturation of the adults (young, middle, and old) living within the family. A continuing search for new models and paradigms is necessary, if nursing is to move substantively from old views of the family as the appendage of the patient to newer studies of the family as an element of human health and adult developmental potential.

Only one published volume was found in nursing that included developmental aspects of family life from the perspective of normal people over the entire family life span (Knafl & Grace, 1978). In this volume, several separate studies were presented. The methodology used in all the studies was indepth interviews using a symbolic interactionist framework. Issues addressed in the interviews included concepts relevant to adult development, such as launching and emancipation from parents, negotiating a division of responsibility between couples, creating interpersonal rules in the new family, establishing a sexual relationship, and developing the rules for extracouple relationships. While these data were interesting and heuristically appealing, there was a disappointing superficiality to their presentation and analysis. The findings were reported through the medium of vignettes and case study quotes that suffer from a lack of predictive interpretation and prescriptive theory building.

Other investigators studied aspects of the marital relationship, including conflict in the marriage (Hoskins, 1979; Hurley, 1981), stabilizing influences of marriage (Kinsler, 1976), and the impact of divorce on the individuals (Peterson, 1978). These phenomena are potentially developmental but were not addressed as such in the research. One study, which at least attended to the wife as adult woman in the family planning process, was conducted by Meleis (1971) who examined the changing self-concept of the woman in relation to the couple's effectiveness in family planning.

The family is an important focus for health/illness research within nursing. The family is a place where adults continue to develop (or not) and, hence the family should become a priority focus for studies of adult life.

WOMEN'S HEALTH—FEMINISM AS A
MATURATIONAL FORCE

Recently, some nurse-researchers have turned their attention to women's health. The literature on this topic was reviewed to assess its philosophical orientation to the study of women as adult human beings in the process of growing and maturing. McBride and McBride's (1981) important caution, that researchers should not continue to study women as if they were no more than female organ systems, is an important benchmark in women's health research. These authors appealed for "non context stripping" orientations to research. This idea is analogous to the point made several times in this chapter about mothers, fathers, and married couples: the woman subject should be studied within the proper context as a maturing, changing adult. McBride and McBride referred to this as studying women's lived experience. Dougherty (1978) was specific in her plea that women's health research on topics such as the climacteric include attention to adaptability and changing developmental needs of the women subjects.

The studies of women's health most prevalent in the nursing literature focused on menstrual experience (Auger, 1967; Dan, 1980; Golub, 1980; Graham, 1980; Kay, 1981; Most, Woods, Dery, & Most, 1981; Voda, 1980, 1981; Woods, Most, & Dery, 1982). There were only a few studies found on menopause (LaRocco & Polit, 1980; Uphold & Susman, 1981). Several investigators studied the impact upon women of health alterations of various kinds (Andersen, 1980; Cosper, Fuller, & Robinson, 1980; Hart, 1967/1968; Putt, 1977a; Williams, 1980; Woods & Earp, 1978; Woods, 1980). In addition, there was a specialized group of studies undertaken by nurses on the effects of rape and abuse upon the later health and emotional development of the victims (Burgess & Holmstrom, 1976a, 1976b; Ipema, 1979).

The studies on women's health will be critiqued in the context of their potential contribution to the science of human development. The investigators in this group were more sensitive and humanistic about studying their respective phenomena than earlier (typically male) biomedical and behavioral researchers have been. Attention was given to rigorous documentation of menstrual cycle experiences rather than relying on one-time recall questions. However, the investigators did not include contextual frameworks about the subjects' developmental stage and maturational progression within that stage. The outcomes would be richer and more insightful if a developmental context were overlaid upon the particular women's health framework.

ILLNESS AS A MATURATIONAL FORCE

Researchers studying illness or crisis in children would not plunge into their research without a thorough knowledge of normal growth and development of infants and children. The same rule now is beginning to apply to research on the elderly; students attend to theory about aging and gerontology as a basis for geriatric or wellness research on the elderly. But no such rules apply in studies of young or middle aged adults. Researchers studying adults are not required to have a base of developmental knowledge about their target populations. There is no rite of passage or educational credentialling required to study adults, or so it would seem when the studies of ill adults are analyzed from a developmental perspective.

The literature about adults under the stress of life change events, situational stresses, accidents, and acute and chronic illnesses of self and family members was reviewed. This search depended on the titles of articles, and thus many studies likely were missed. The titles chosen for review contained terms that implied attention to key concepts of adult life. Unfortunately, the research designs did not incorporate developmental variables. There were many studies of adult subjects who were undergoing a variety of illness experiences or life change events (Bell, 1977; Erickson & Swain, 1982; Hogue, 1974; Kennell, Slyter, & Klaus, 1970; McNeil & Pesznecker, 1977; Parker, 1981; Pesznecker & McNeil, 1975; Rosen & Bibring, 1968; Stember, 1977; Williams & Nikolaisen, 1982; Wolff, Nielson, & Schiller, 1970). Usually chronological age was mentioned as a straightforward demographic variable that did not show significance in the data analysis, perhaps because mean ages rather than developmental age groupings were used. Two investigators focused on the specific maturational crisis of caring for elderly parents (Archbold, 1980; Lepper, 1968). While the topic was inherently maturational (elderly parent caring), the theoretical approach taken was situational and involved a listing of ramifications (mostly negative) for the middle-aged adult. However, some developmental issues arose, for example, the issues of commitment and responsibility to kin (Archbold, 1980) and the reexperiencing of unresolved conflicts between mother (elderly-ill) and daughter (middle-aged) caretaker.

Chronic illness research is an area of high potential compatibility with research on adult development. Particularly relevant are chronic illnesses that require permanent lifestyle change. The studies reviewed in this area did not include a theoretical grounding in adult development (Cohen, Wallston, & Wallston, 1976; Putt, 1977b; Reed, 1970; Wang, Zeitz, Schwartz, & Goss, 1962; Woods & Hulka, 1979). Investigators rarely differentiated between or among decades of adulthood, and when they did the age spans were not given any substantive attention. A grounding in adult development would dictate a conceptually grounded separate analysis of persons in young adulthood from those in middle adulthood, but this type of analysis was not found.

From a developmental frame of reference, it is logical that a ± 25-year-old chronically ill or disabled person is assaulted at the peak of physical development and is faced with disruption in the early development of work life, (new) family life, and emerging community participation. On the other hand, the ± 45-year-old chronically ill or disabled person is faced with responsibility for schoolage or adolescent children, economic commitments (mortgage or equivalent), occupational responsibilities (managerial or informal leader), aging parents, and community positions (e.g., scout leader, Sunday school teacher). Persons in different adult stages may not show quantitative differences in their response to illness, but attention to qualitative and contextual differences are equally important. Indeed, such differences could have ramifications for the building of prescriptive theories for nursing practice.

Catanzaro (1980) conducted a study of 126 persons with urinary bladder dysfunction secondary to multiple sclerosis. Her goal was to determine the effects of bladder dysfunction on the subjects' accomplishment of the developmental tasks of their respective adult stage. She used indepth interviews and found that all four major areas of adult life (work, family, community, and self) were negatively affected. Work and leisure experiences decreased markedly. The ability to remain employed was highly threatened. The marital and parenting tasks also were affected; most subjects had either divorced, separated, or had no sexual relationship with the spouse if still sharing an abode. Relationships with children deteriorated since the parent felt more immature (not toilet trained) than the children and in this context felt unable to act as a role model for the children. Nearly all of the 126 subjects had stopped engaging in community activities such as attendance at church or social functions. The result was an insular lifestyle, deteriorating self-concept, and fixation on the urinary incontinence and the scheduling/care that its management entailed. Catanzaro concluded that the adult development of these persons was greatly retarded and characterized their lifestyles as "shamefully different."

This study was a unique discovery in the search process to construct this chapter. One hopes that Catanzaro's study will provide the impetus for further investigation. Eventually, a set of nursing interventions could be developed to prevent or reverse the negative impact that chronic conditions can have on adult development and family life.

COMMUNITY LIFE AS A MATURATIONAL FORCE

Brandt and Weinert (1981) developed a Personal Resource Questionnaire to measure social support in chronic illness. Several developmental issues were encompassed by the concept of social support. These included aspects of friendship, familiazation, and community participation and their impact on the individual's sense of worth, sense of being loved, and self-esteem. One part of the instrument specifically included items about intimacy, social integration, nurturance, and self-worth, all of which are developmental concepts. The report on validity and reliability (using 149 spouses of persons with multiple sclerosis) showed careful evaluation of the instrument's psychometric properties. Additional work must be done, of course, but this intrument would appear to have utility for the study of adults within the context of social participation/social support. It is unfortunate that the authors did not incorporate a developmental perspective. However, it would be a relatively straightforward matter to incorporate a developmental perspective in the use and analysis of the Personal Resource Questionnaire.

Stevenson (1982) developed the Margin in Life Scale to operationalize McClusky's (1963) adult development construct of

$$\frac{\text{Load}}{\text{Power}} = \text{Margin in Life}$$

The scale has six subscales, which correspond to major dimensions of adult life: self concept, body/physical health, spirituality/religiosity, family, extrafamilial relationships (e.g., work, leisure, friendships, social networking), and nonperson environment (e.g., taxes, real estate, weather, neighborhood, laws, and crime). The basis of McClusky's construct is that there is a ratio in life between all the sources of power (energy) to conduct one's internal and external life processes and all the sources of load (uses of the energy). The sources of power (energy sources) should outweigh the sources of load (drains of energy), and this unequal ratio produces a margin which is available to accept new stimuli such as additional commitments in life or to cope with crises. The psychometric properties of the Margin in Life Scale have been investigated using normal adult volunteers aged 20 to 70 (Stevenson, 1982) and with various older adult groups (Stevenson, 1980). Much additional validity and reliability work remains to be done, but the scale could be useful for the study of the perceived quality of adult life under various conditions of normalcy and crisis.

SITUATIONAL CHANGES OF ADULTHOOD

There are situational changes in adult life that occur primarily in one stage or age range. Nurse researchers have done studies on these situational issues. Retirement is an age-related situational change that is forced upon adults in western society by virtue of social understandings of and expectations for the aging person. A few sources were found on the impact of retirement (Cassels, Eckstein, & Fortinash, 1981; Heller, Walsh, & Wilson, 1981), but they did not include consideration of the effect of retirement on adult development.

Another topic that has received attention by nurses is death of the spouse and the ensuing bereavement process (Constantino, 1981; Demi, 1978; Dracup & Breu, 1978; Hampe, 1975; McCorkle, 1977; Saunders, 1981). These studies were based in a developmental stage. That is, the death of the spouse is most typically the experience of persons in their new middle years or later adult years. The investigators used a variety of theoretical premises but did not attend to adult development. However, emotional growth is a potential byproduct of the grief and loss experience. Thus research attention should be directed to effects of bereavement beyond the immediate period of grieving.

Finally, one study was reviewed in which the investigators looked at a common human experience in terms of its developmental meaning. Johnston, Fitzpatrick, and Donovan (1982) studied the relative influence of developmental stage and depression on the experience of time among healthy adults. They hypothesized that developmental stage would be a better predictor of time sense than depression, sex, or marital status. They found that developmental stage was a more significant factor on eight of the nine temporal variables and concluded that there is support for the developmentally based nature of temporality. A developmental approach also may be useful for research on other holistic concepts of human experience such as movement, rhythm, or sound perception.

PROMISE FOR THE FUTURE

An understanding of the multiple issues and tasks of adulthood gives rise to a myriad of research questions about health, higher-level wellness, stress, acute and chronic health problems, and other events that impinge upon health. The occurrence of health problems is both an overlay upon the already complex mission of adult life and simultaneously an additional stimulus for enhancing emotional maturation. Thus, a fertile field for research and theory building is provided by the constant interplay between health crises and developmental processes. Since the research on adult development from a nursing/health care perspective is so sparse, a model is suggested to encourage work in this area; this model should be considered illustrative rather than exhaustive. It is meant to enhance rather than discourage the creativity of fertile minds.

Figure 1 shows a systematized matrix of potential areas for productive research by nurses and others in the health field. Across the bottom of the figure, age groupings are displayed. The three age groups of particular interest here are young adulthood, the core middle years, and the new

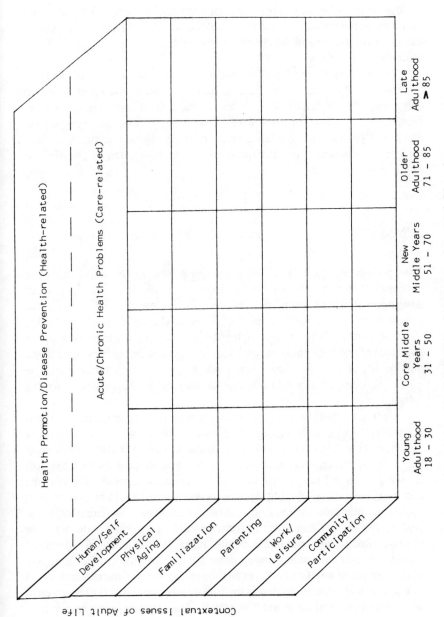

Figure 1.   Model for Nursing Research on Adulthood.

middle years. The two stages of older adulthood, referred to in some literature as the young-old and the old-old, are included simply to complete the life cycle and to highlight the appropriateness of developmental research on the elderly.

The left side of the figure contains a list of contextual issues of adult life that already receive considerable nursing research attention. The two categories shown across the top are health-related and care-related research. Health-related research would include studies on disease prevention and health promotion; care-related research refers to the traditional nursing focus of illness care. Research questions can be stimulated by focusing on any cell in the matrix.

SUMMARY

This review included the diverse nursing literature on adults with the expectation that it should contain theoretical underpinnings about adult development. In selecting the studies, the reviewer faced a dilemma: review only that literature (about half dozen studies) that clearly identified itself as coming from a developmental perspective, or review a broad spectrum of research on adults and point out the consistent blind spot in the nursing literature. The choice was made to pursue the latter course. The goal of this chapter is not to criticize the past but to chart a course for the future.

During the next decade, nurse researchers should engage in constructing theory about adulthood, especially as the dynamics of crisis, illness, or higher-level wellness impact on adult development. Attention also should be given to the reciprocal issue of developmental progress (or lack thereof) showing a causal linkage with the onset of crises or illnesses. Further, the complex interactions of adult developmental stages should receive at least contextual attention in traditional nursing topics such as parent-child research, family health/stress research, research on coping with acute or chronic illness, and women's health research. "Contextual attention" means a theoretically sound appreciation for the maturational forces at play in any sample of adult subjects, even though the focus of the research is not developmental. One hopes that in the future, basic attention will be given to adult developmental stage and that growth issues will underpin research on a myriad of topics.

REFERENCES

Aguilera, D. C., Messick, J. M., & Farrell, M. S. Maturational crises. In D. C. Aguilera & J. M. Messick (Eds.), *Crisis intervention: Theory and methodology*. St. Louis: Mosby, 1970

Andersen, M. D. Health needs of drug dependent clients: Focus on women. *Women and Health,* 1980, *5,* 23–33.

Archbold, P. G. Impact of parent caring on middle-aged offspring. *Journal of Gerontological Nursing,* 1980, *6,* 78–85.

Auger, J. A. R. A psychophysiological study of the normal menstrual cycle and of some possible effects of oral contraceptives (Doctoral dissertation, University of California, 1967). *Dissertation Abstracts,* 1967, *28,* 3070B–3071B. (University Microfilms No. 67-17, 356)

Bell, J. M. Stressful life events and coping methods in mental illness and wellness behaviors. *Nursing Research,* 1977, *26,* 136–141.

Bornstein, R. Cognitive and psycho-social development in middlescence. In C. S. Schuster & S. S. Ashburn (Eds.), *The process of human development.* Boston: Little, Brown, 1980.

Bowen, S. M., & Miller, B. C. Paternal attachment behavior as related to presence at delivery and preparenthood classes: A pilot study. *Nursing Research,* 1980, *29,* 307–311.

Brandt, P. A., & Weinert, C. The PRQ—A social support measure. *Nursing Research,* 1981, *30,* 277–280.

Burgess, A. W., & Holmstrom, L. L. Coping behaviors and the rape victim. *American Journal of Psychiatry,* 1976, *133,* 413–417. (a)

Burgess, A. W., & Holmstrom, L. L. Rape: Its effect on task performance at varying stages in the life cycle. In M. J. Walker & S. L. Brodsky (Eds.), *Sexual assault.* Lexington, Mass.: Lexington Books, 1976. (b)

Cassels, C. S., Eckstein, A. M., & Fortinash, K. M. Retirement: Aspects, response, and nursing implications. *Journal of Gerontological Nursing,* 1981, *7,* 355–359.

Catanzaro, M. Shamefully different: A personal meaning of urinary bladder dysfunction (Doctoral dissertation, Union for Experimenting Colleges and Universities–West, San Francisco, 1980). *Dissertation Abstracts International,* 1980, *42,* 4166A. (University Microfilms No. DA8204984)

Cohen, B. D., Wallston, B. S., & Wallston, K. A. Sex counseling in cardiac rehabilitation. *Archives of Physical Medicine and Rehabilitation,* 1976, *57,* 473–474.

Constantino, R. E. Bereavement crisis intervention for widows in grief and mourning. *Nursing Research,* 1981, *30,* 351–353.

Cosper, B., Fuller, S., & Robinson, G. J. Characteristics of posthospital recovery following hysterectomy. In A. J. Dan, E. A. Graham, & C. P. Beecher (Eds.), *The menstrual cycle: A synthesis of interdisciplinary research* (Vol. 1). New York: Springer, 1980.

Cronenwett, L. R. Father participation in child care: A critical review. *Research in Nursing and Health,* 1982, *5,* 63–72.

Cronenwett, L. R., & Newmark, L. L. Fathers' responses to childbirth. *Nursing Research,* 1974, *23,* 210–217.

Dan, A. J. Free-associative versus self-report measures of emotional change over the menstrual cycle. In A. J. Dan, E. A. Graham, & C. P. Beecher (Eds.), *The menstrual cycle: A synthesis of interdisciplinary research* (Vol. 1). New York: Springer, 1980.

Demi, A. S. Adjustment to widowhood after a sudden death: Suicide and non-suicide survivors compared. In M. V. Batey (Ed.), *Communicating nursing research* (Vol. 11). Boulder, Colo.: Western Interstate Commission for Higher Education, 1978.

Dennis, K. E. A man and a woman in the middle years. *Journal of Gerontological Nursing,* 1981, *7,* 417–422.

Diekelmann, N. L. Emotional tasks of the middle adult. *American Journal of Nursing,* 1975, *75,* 997–1000.

Diekelmann, N. L. The young adult. *American Journal of Nursing,* 1976, *76,* 1272–1289.

Donaldson, S. K., & Crowley, D. M. The discipline of nursing. *Nursing Outlook,* 1978, *26,* 113–126.

Dougherty, M. C. An anthropological perspective on aging and women in the middle years. In E. E. Bauwens (Ed.), *The anthropology of health.* St. Louis: Mosby, 1978.

Dracup, K. A., & Breu, C. S. Using nursing research findings to meet the needs of grieving spouses. *Nursing Research,* 1978, *27,* 212–216.

Draheim, B. B., & Ashburn, S. S. Biophysical and cognitive development in young adulthood. In C. S. Schuster & S. S. Ashburn (Eds.), *The process of human development.* Boston: Little, Brown, 1980.

Duvall, E. M. *Family development* (3rd ed.). Philadelphia: Lippincott, 1967.

Ebersole, P., & Hess, P. *Toward healthy aging.* St. Louis: Mosby, 1981.

Erickson, H., & Swain, M. A. A model for assessing potential adaptation to stress. *Research in Nursing and Health,* 1982, *5,* 93–101.

Golub, S. Premenstrual changes in mood, personality, and cognitive function. In A. J. Dan, E. A. Graham, & C. P. Beecher (Eds.), *The menstrual cycle: A synthesis of interdisciplinary research* (Vol. 1). New York: Springer, 1980.

Graham, E. A. Cognition as related to menstrual cycle phase and estrogen level. In A. J. Dan, E. A. Graham, & C. P. Beecher (Eds.), *The menstrual cycle: A synthesis of interdisciplinary research* (Vol. 1). New York: Springer, 1980.

Gruis, M. Beyond maternity: Postpartum concerns of mothers. *MCN, American Journal of Maternal Child Nursing,* 1977, *2,* 182–188.

Hall, J. E. Growth: A transcending experience. In J. E. Hall & B. R. Weaver (Eds.), *Nursing of families in crisis.* Philadelphia: Lippincott, 1974.

Hampe, S. O. Needs of the grieving spouse in a hospital setting. *Nursing Research,* 1975, *24,* 113–120.

Hanson, S. Single custodial fathers and the parent-child relationship. *Nursing Research,* 1981, *30,* 202–204.

Hargreaves, A. G. Making the most of the middle years. *MCN, American Journal of Nursing,* 1975, *75,* 1772–1776.

Hart, M. S. The relationship between reported satisfaction with body image, anxiety, and the occurrence of physiological deviations among healthy college-age females (Doctoral dissertation, New York University, 1967). *Dissertation Abstracts*, 1968, *28*, 4376A–4377A. (University Microfilms No. 68-4778)

Heller, B. R., Walsh, F. J., & Wilson, K. M. Seniors helping seniors: Training older adults as new personnel resources in home health care. *Journal of Gerontological Nursing*, 1981, *7*, 552–555.

Hogue, C. C. Coping resources, stress and health change in middle age (Doctoral dissertation, University of North Carolina, 1974). *Dissertation Abstracts International*, 1974, *35*, 4017B–4018B. (University Microfilms No. 75–4828)

Hoskins, C. N. Level of activation, body temperature, and interpersonal conflict in family relationships. *Nursing Research*, 1979, *28*, 154–160.

Hurley, P. M. Communication patterns and conflict in marital dyads. *Nursing Research*, 1981, *30*, 38–42.

Ipema, D. K. Rape: The process of recovery. *Nursing Research*, 1979, *28*, 272–275.

Johnston, R. L., Fitzpatrick, J. J., & Donovan, M. J. Developmental stage: Relationship to temporal dimensions. *Nursing Research*, 1982, *31*, 120. (Abstract)

Kay, M. A. Meanings of menstruation to Mexican American women. In P. Komnenich, M. McSweeney, J. A. Noack, & N. Elder (Eds.), *The menstrual cycle: Research and implications for women's health* (Vol. 2). New York: Springer, 1981.

Kennell, J. H., Slyter, H., & Klaus, M. H. The mourning response of parents to the death of a newborn infant. *New England Journal of Medicine*, 1970, *283*, 344–349.

Kessler, E. R. Comparative analysis of distress among mothers of hospitalized two through four year old children and the relationship to social class membership (Doctoral dissertation, New York University, 1969). *Dissertation Abstracts International*, 1969, *30*, 2771B–2772B. (University Microfilms No. 69–21, 215)

Kinsler, D. D. Life style: Marital stability versus the swinging singles existence. *Journal of Psychiatric Nursing and Mental Health Services*, 1976, *14*(9), 20–21.

Knafl, K. A., & Grace, H. K. (Eds.). *Families across the life cycle*. Boston: Little, Brown, 1978.

Kunst-Wilson, W., & Cronenwett, L. Nursing care for the emerging family: Promoting paternal behavior. *Research in Nursing and Health*, 1981, *4*, 201–211.

LaRocco, S. A., & Polit, D. F. Women's knowledge about the menopause. *Nursing Research*, 1980, *29*, 10–13.

Larsen, V. L. Stresses of the childbearing years. *American Journal of Public Health*, 1966, *56*, 32–36.

Lepper, K. E. Problems and coping patterns of the household member caring for the adult female cancer patient in the home (Doctoral dissertation, Columbia University, 1968). *Dissertation Abstracts*, 1968, *29*, 2442A. (University Microfilms No. 69–667)

Martinson, I. M. Loss of a child: Two case studies. In D. K. Kjervik & I. M.

Martinson (Eds.), *Women in stress: A nursing perspective*. New York: Apple-ton-Century-Crofts, 1979.

Martinson, I. M., & Jorgens, C. Reports of a parent support group. In I. M. Martinson (Ed.), *Home care for the dying child: Professional and family perspectives*. New York: Appleton-Century-Crofts, 1976.

May, K. A. A typology of detachment/involvement styles adopted during pregnancy by first-time expectant fathers. *Western Journal of Nursing Research*, 1980, *2*, 445–453.

McBride, A. B., & McBride, W. L. Theoretical underpinnings for women's health. *Women and Health*, 1981, *6*, 37–55.

McCaffery, M., & Johnson, D. E. Effect of parent group discussion upon epistemic responses. *Nursing Research*, 1967, *16*, 352–358.

McClusky, H. Y. The course of the adult life span. In W. C. Hallenbeck (Ed.), *Psychology of adults*. Washington, D. C.: Adult Education of the U.S.A., 1963.

McCorkle, R. Terminal illness: Human attachments and intended goals. In M. V. Batey (Ed.), *Communicating nursing research* (Vol. 9). Boulder, Colo.: Western Interstate Commission for Higher Education, 1977.

McNeil, J., & Pesznecker, B. L. Keeping people well despite life change crises. *Public Health Reports*, 1977, *92*, 343–348.

Meleis, A. I. Self-concept and family planning. *Nursing Research*, 1971, *20*, 229–236.

Mercer, R. T. A theoretical framework for studying factors that impact on the maternal role. *Nursing Research*, 1981, *30*, 73–77.

Merrow, D. L., & Johnson, B. S. Perceptions of the mother's role with her hospitalized child. *Nursing Research*, 1968, *17*, 155–156.

Most, A., Woods, N. F., Dery, G. K., & Most, B. Distress associated with menstruation among Israeli women. *International Journal of Nursing Studies*, 1981, *18*, 61–71.

Mourad, L. A. Biophysical development during middlescence. In C. S. Schuster & S. S. Ashburn (Eds.), *The process of human development*. Boston: Little, Brown, 1980.

Nikolaisen, S. M., & Williams, R. A. Parents' view of support following the loss of their infant to sudden infant death syndrome. *Western Journal of Nursing Research*, 1980, *2*, 593–601.

Norbeck, J. S., & Sheiner, M. Sources of social support related to single-parent functioning. *Research in Nursing and Health*, 1982, *5*, 3–11.

Palermo, E. Remarriage: Parental perceptions of steprelations with children and adolescents. *Journal of Psychiatric Nursing and Mental Health Services*, 1980, *18*(4), 9–13.

Parker, K. P. Anxiety and complications in patients on hemodialysis. *Nursing Research*, 1981, *30*, 334–336.

Pesznecker, B. L., & McNeil, J. Relationship among health habits, social assets, psychologic well-being, life change and alterations in health status. *Nursing Research*, 1975, *24*, 442–447.

Peterson, L. C. Guilt, attribution of responsibility and resolution of the divorce crisis. *Image*, 1978, *10*, 57. (Abstract)

Putt, A. M. Effects of noise on fatigue in healthy middle-aged adults. In M. V.

Batey (Ed.), *Communicating nursing research* (Vol. 8). Boulder, Colo.: Western Interstate Commission for Higher Education, 1977. (a)

Putt, A. M. Patterns of response to a prescribed exercise in middle-aged diabetic subjects. In M. V. Batey (Ed.), *Communicating nursing research* (Vol. 10). Boulder, Colo.: Western Interstate Commission for Higher Education, 1977. (b)

Reed, D. L. Social disengagement in chronically ill patients. *Nursing Research,* 1970, *19,* 109–115.

Reiber, V. Is the nurturing role natural to fathers? *MCN, The American Journal of Maternal Child Nursing,* 1976, *1,* 366–371.

Rosen, J. L., & Bibring, G. L. Psychological reactions of hospitalized male patients to a heart attack: Age and social-class differences. In B. L. Neugarten (Ed.), *Middle age and aging.* Chicago: University of Chicago Press, 1968.

Rubin, R. Attainment of the maternal role: Part 1. Processes. *Nursing Research,* 1967, *16,* 237–245. (a)

Rubin, R. Attainment of the maternal role: Part II. Models and referents. *Nursing Research,* 1967, *16,* 342–346. (b)

Saunders, J. M. A process of bereavement resolution: Uncoupled identity. *Western Journal of Nursing Research,* 1981, *3,* 319–336.

Skipper, J. K., Leonard, R. C., & Rhymes, J. Child hospitalization and social interaction: An experimental study of mothers' feelings of stress, adaptation and satisfaction. *Medical Care,* 1968, *6,* 496–506.

Smith, M. E. P. Maturational crisis of pregnancy: Associated themes and problems (Doctoral dissertation, Boston University, 1965). *Dissertation Abstracts,* 1967, *28,* 3354B–3355B. (University Microfilms No. 66–1397)

Stember, M. L. Familial response to hospitalization of an adult member. In M. V. Batey (Ed.), *Communicating nursing research* (Vol. 9). Boulder, Colo.: Western Interstate Commission for Higher Education, 1977.

Stern, P. N. Affiliating in stepfather families: Teachable strategies leading to stepfather-child friendship. *Western Journal of Nursing Research,* 1982, *4,* 75–89.

Stevenson, J. S. *Issues and crises during middlescence.* New York: Appleton-Century-Crofts, 1977.

Stevenson, J. S. Load, power and margin in older adults. *Geriatric Nursing,* 1980, *1,* 52–55.

Stevenson, J. S. Construction of a scale to measure load, power, and margin in life. *Nursing Research,* 1982, *31,* 222–225.

Thomas, B. C. The maturing teenage mother. *Women and Health,* 1979, *4,* 147–157.

Uphold, C. R., & Susman, E. J. Self-reported climacteric symptoms as a function of the relationships between marital adjustment and childrearing stage. *Nursing Research,* 1981, *30,* 84–88.

Voda, A. Pattern of progesterone and aldosterone in ovulating women during the menstrual cycle. In A. J. Dan, E. A. Graham, & C. P. Beecher (Eds.), *The menstrual cycle: A synthesis of interdisciplinary research* (Vol. 1). New York: Springer, 1980.

Voda, A. Alterations of the menstrual cycle: Hormonal and mechanical. In P. Komnenich, M. McSweeney, J. A. Noack, & N. Elder (Eds.), *The menstrual cycle: Research and implications for women's health* (Vol. 2). New York: Springer, 1981.

Wang, M., Zeitz, L., Schwartz, D., & Goss, M. Study of nursing needs of the chronically ill. *Nursing Research*, 1962, *11*, 236–237.

Williams, F. S. Intervention in maturational crises. In J. E. Hall & B. R. Weaver (Eds.), *Nursing of families in crisis*. Philadelphia: Lippincott, 1974.

Williams, M. A. Cultural factors and hysterectomy. In A. J. Dan, E. A. Graham, & C. P. Beecher (Eds.), *The menstrual cycle: A synthesis of interdisciplinary research* (Vol. 1). New York: Springer, 1980.

Williams, R. A., & Nikolaisen, S. M. Sudden infant death syndrome: Parents' responses to the loss of their infant. *Research in Nursing and Health*, 1982, *5*, 55–61.

Willmuth, R., Weaver, L., & Borenstein, J. Satisfaction with prepared childbirth and locus of control. *Journal of Obstetric, Gynecologic and Neonatal Nursing*, 1978, *7*(3), 33–37.

Wolff, J. R., Nielson, P. E., & Schiller, P. The emotional reaction to a stillbirth. *American Journal of Obstetrics and Gynecology*, 1970, *108*, 73–77.

Woods, N. F. Women's roles and illness episodes: A prospective study. *Research in Nursing and Health*, 1980, *3*, 137–145.

Woods, N. F., & Earp, J. L. Women with cured breast cancer. *Nursing Research*, 1978, *27*, 279–285.

Woods, N. F., & Hulka, B. S. Symptom reports and illness behavior among employed women and homemakers. *Journal of Community Health*, 1979, *5*, 36–45.

Woods, N. F., Most, A., & Dery, G. K. Estimating perimenstrual distress: A comparison of two methods. *Research in Nursing and Health*, 1982, *5*, 81–91.

CHAPTER 4

Clinical Geriatric Nursing Research

MARY OPAL WOLANIN
COLLEGE OF NURSING
UNIVERSITY OF ARIZONA

CONTENTS

This review of clinical geriatric nursing research covers the 30 years, 1952 to 1982, that coincide with the era of nursing research journals and journals of gerontological/geriatric nursing (1975 to 1982). Early in the period covered, there were few studies in the care of the elderly, but at this time a number of nurses are choosing clinical research in this area. There have been few funded studies in clinical geriatric nursing, and much of the published research has been that which met requirements for graduate degrees in nursing. At this time there is a turning point: clinical studies are increasing in number and quality, and there are more opportunities to publish in refereed journals. There are excellent means of retrieval through computerized searches and the *Cumulative Index to Nursing and Allied Health Literature, International Nursing Index,* and *Index Medicus.* The future promises a productive and exciting era for clinical geriatric nursing research. This chapter recounts the prologue.

DEFINITIONS

The person who attempts to review clinical geriatric nursing research is faced with the problems of definitions. When nursing itself lacks a firm definition, and the other terms have subjective meanings, it is necessary to start with definitions of the terms used in this chapter.

Clinical geriatric nursing research has been defined by MacRae (Note 1). "Our business is nursing. Therefore our clinical research will be focused on nursing action. Our testing of nursing theories and others' theories used in nursing will be carried out in relation to elders—their needs for services; their resources for well-being, their responses to health related interventions" (p. 1). The basis of nursing theories is nursing concepts and nursing hypotheses. The purpose is an increase in the quality of patient care by understanding, productivity, and direction. Clinical research begins with observation and questions, and although it becomes very abstract in conceptualization, it remains relevant to practice (MacRae, Note 1). Investigators must conceptualize clinical nursing research in such a way as to develop researchable questions. These must be addressed by practitioner and researcher alike if priorities in clinical nursing research are to be identified.

Geriatric nursing and *gerontological nursing* are often confused. Clinical geriatric nursing is the preferred term for this review, for it is concerned primarily with the health of the older person. This involves maintenance of health, prevention of illness and disability, and the care of the ill, leading to restoration of health when possible or to a peaceful death. It draws on knowledge of the total life span, which has been prologue to this time of life, and is inextricably bound to any consideration of the health of the aged person. Geriatric nursing relies on the body of knowledge known as gerontology for information about the process of aging, drawn from the biophysical, psychosocial, and socioeconomic factors impinging on the person.

Gerontology is the study of aging. Nursing gerontology includes the definition of gerontology, geriatrics (medical treatment of old age and its diseases), geriatric nursing, and nursing research (Gunter & Miller, 1977). The clinical studies reviewed here fall into the narrower category of geriatric nursing rather than the broader scope of gerontological nursing.

The first criterion used in selection of studies to be reviewed is that the research must meet MacRae's (Note 1) definition of clinical research. The second criterion is that the study must be accessible to the reader. Nursing research journals, geriatric/gerontological nursing journals, and doctoral dissertations were reviewed for studies that met the first criterion. Studies used included a clearly stated, researchable question, a systematic collection of data, analysis of data, and stated conclusions. Implications for nursing were not always stated.

PREVIOUS REVIEWS

Four reviews were done of gerontological nursing literature dating from the year 1952 to the present. Although each report differed in focus, the four reports showed trends, and the history of gerontological/geriatric nursing can be read from them.

The Basson Report (1955 to 1966)

A review of the nursing literature in the care of the aged by Brown, Basson, and Burchett (1967) was the basis for the Basson report (1967). She summarized the nursing literature by saying that a large scale review was similar to research in that there were educated guesses about trends, and that relationships became the basis for predictions and hypotheses. The report was generally based on nonresearch articles. Nevertheless some were fact finding, descriptive, and empirical and provided the basis and direction for gerontological research to grow (Brimmer, 1979). Basson included a breakdown of the literature by title, journal citation, and type of study in chart form. Of the 438 articles about nursing and the aged, only fifty-two were concerned with research. There was a paucity of theory development. Much emphasis was placed on depersonalization, dependency, infection, incontinence, diabetes, and deformities.

The Gunter-Miller Overview (1951 to 1976)

Gunter and Miller (1977) presented a comprehensive survey of nursing gerontology in the research context of social and medical gerontology and the state of the research art itself. Articles published in *Nursing Research* from its first issue in 1952 to 1976 were the principal source of nursing research in the overview. Nursing studies were summarized and nursing issues identified. The overview indicated only five clinical studies during the late 1960s (Adams, 1966; Grosicki, 1968; Neely & Patrick, 1968; Stotsky & Rhetts, 1966; Van Drimmelen & Rollins, 1969). There were many studies during the 1970s, but only four reflected a clinical interest (Ankenbrandt & Tanner, 1971; Baltes & Zerbe, 1976; DeWalt, 1975; Managan, 1974).

Gunter and Miller (1977) isolated psychosocial studies from clinical research but divided the research into three areas: (a) psychosocial needs and characteristics of the elderly, (b) attitudes of caregivers, and (c) intervention and treatment approaches to meet the psychosocial needs of the elderly. Nursing intervention research (Carlson, 1968; Carpenter & Simon, 1960; Grosicki, 1968) was included in the nursing concerns of this chapter.

In addition to the overview of research, Gunter and Miller (1977) analyzed the research issues. They found problems in methodology, such as the need for longitudinal studies rather than cross-sectional studies, and problems with comparing studies due to dissimilar sampling on the basis of age, health, and other variables. The general lack of clinical research was mentioned, while specific areas such as management of patients with chronic problems, especially those with chronic brain disease, were emphasized. Research utilization by the practitioner was an important need.

The Brimmer Review (1979)

Brimmer selected three time periods, 1966, 1971, and 1976, as the basis for her review. This expanded the base to the 150 nursing journals reviewed in the *International Nursing Index,* which was used as the source of the citations, and the nonnursing journals reviewed by the *Index Medicus.* Only American publications were used in a chart in which articles were classified according to subject area (geriatric dentistry, geriatric nursing, aged, aging, and rehabilitation, etc.). Geriatric nursing citations increased in the *International Nursing Index* from two in 1966 to 114 in 1976. Brimmer was concerned primarily with nursing research in the context of funding agencies, nursing educational systems, multidisciplinary research teams, and social and health care systems; she made no attempt to describe or evaluate the research cited. She recommended that researchers be politically astute, aware of trends in the social system and the health care system, and that they develop skills in working with multidisciplinary teams. As had Gunter and Miller (1977), Brimmer saw the need for utilization of research in the clinical area.

The Kayser-Jones Report (1981)

Surveying *Western Journal of Nursing Research, Research in Nursing and Health, Journal of Gerontological Research,* and *Geriatric Nursing* from beginning dates of publication through July 1980, and *Nursing Research* from January 1977 to July 1980, Kayser-Jones found forty-four articles that dealt with gerontological nursing. Twelve of these forty-four articles dealt with a clinical research focus, but these were not cited. Her conclusions were that there were limitations of breadth and scope of the reported research and that there appeared to be no large scale, well defined research programs that systematically investigated prevention, promotion, maintenance, and restoration of health for the elderly. Like Brimmer (1979), Kayser-Jones considered the educational context in which gerontological nursing research was done. The lack of gerontological and geriatric nursing content in the basic nursing educational programs leads to a lack of preparation in this field for research at the graduate level. The first need is for introduction of content at all levels and for development of faculty to teach the care of the elderly. The second is to stimulate research in the nursing care of the elderly so it will lead to making quality health care available to them.

To summarize the four reviews (Basson, 1967; Brimmer, 1979; Gunter & Miller, 1977; Kayser-Jones, 1981), it can be said that although their materials overlapped, they were not coterminous. They offer a background on the development of geriatric clinical nursing research, the context in which it was done, and its direction at that time. Only Gunter and Miller (1977) summarized the methodology and the findings of the clinical nursing studies that were cited. Lack of clinical studies was an issue throughout the overviews, and the lack of preparation of the practitioner, faculty, and researcher was a common concern.

FACTORS IDENTIFIED FOR INVESTIGATION

Personal Care

Nursing has always been associated with taking over the self-care function, which illness or disability prevents the individual from performing. Research in this area focused on comfort (Lamb, 1979), foot care (King, 1978; Schank, 1977), oral hygiene (DeWalt, 1975; Van Drimmelen & Rollins, 1969), and skin care, the last more frequently referred to as tissue trauma (Gerber & Van Ort, 1979; Hayter & McPhetridge, 1976; Steadman, Schenk, & Walker, 1980; Verhonick, 1961).

Comfort for the elderly person with hip fracture may consist of being able to lie in the right position. Lamb (1979) found that 50 percent of the patients with hip fracture repairs chose to lie on the affected side. Those lying on the side opposite their usual sleep position were more likely to need analgesia.

Foot problems of the elderly were surveyed by Schank (1977) with a finding that of those 60 persons investigated, 88.76 percent of the women and 61.11 percent of the men had foot problems. Those in the 70 to 79 age group had the most problems. The majority, including those with circulatory disease, cut their own nails, although toenail problems were very common. King (1978) developed a foot assessment tool. Twenty nurses independently examined the feet of 41 clients with the tool. Overall, instrument reliabilty was not assessed; reliability coefficients were determined for each of the 47 items. There was 65 to 95 percent agreement on seventy-four percent of the items. Lack of agreement was found in such items as location of posterior tibial pulse and dorsalis pedis pulse and the color of nails.

Oral care, which included evaluation of the traditional lemon and glycerine solution for mouth care for the dependent elderly as compared to normal saline, was studied by Van Drimmelen and Rollins (1969). Both solutions made important differences in the oral condition from Day 1 to Day 2, but the conclusion drawn was that this related to having oral care at least once a day rather than to the specific agent used. DeWalt (1975) studied the effect of timed hygienic measures on oral mucosa, using a toothbrush or a commercial product called a "toothette." Care was given every four hours during the day to 48 nursing home patients. The toothbrush was more effective in removal of debris and stimulation of gingival tissue but was more traumatic to tissue. In both studies, the investigators found that when oral care was omitted, the mouth quickly reverted to its original state.

Tissue trauma was investigated through the use of nursing intervention to prevent or heal decubitus ulcers. Verhonick (1961) developed a systematic observation checklist for describing tissue trauma and a nursing diagnosis checklist for assessing the physiological condition of the patient in whom trauma occurred. Reducing the occurrence of decubitus ulcers was studied by Steadman, Schenk, and Walker (1980) by decreasing pressure levels under the resting body. They found a stable mattress better for self-care (turning) than a "bouncy" surface. Gerber and Van Ort (1979) tested the use of topical insulin as a method of healing decubitus with results that indicated a strong trend in favor of the use of topical insulin. Using an experimental design, Hayter and McPhetridge (1976) studied a control group that used decubitus cleaning daily and an experimental group with similar treatment but with an added koraya gum ring. After 12 weeks, there was no significant difference in the two methods. A recent Delphi study (Brower & Christ, Note 2) in 59 nursing homes and 40 home health care agencies identified prevention, formation, and treatment of decubiti as the most important type of research for patient welfare in long term care. Tissue trauma continues to present a prevention and treatment challenge to nurses. Experimental research requires an instrument for three-dimensional measuring of healing in tissue trauma. A good assessment instrument for measuring condition of the mouth, its ability to perform biting, chewing, swallowing, and speaking has yet to be developed and is necessary for more research on oral care. Care of feet requires more study in which nursing interventions are tested.

Sleep

Sleep in the hospitalized and nonhospitalized persons aged 60 to 82 years was studied by Pacini and Fitzpatrick (1982). Using 19 persons in each group, differences were found in relation to nocturnal sleep time, other sleep time, bedtime, and awakening. Data analysis pointed to the fact that state of mind, fatigue, and state of health, rather than hospitalization itself, contributed to the greater sleep disturbance found in the hospitalized group. The Sleep Pattern Questionnaire (Baekeland & Hartmann, (1971) and the Sleep Chart (Lewis & Masterson, 1957) were used. There was no assessment of reliability of either instrument; validity of the Sleep Pattern Questionnaire was assessed.

Dittmar and Dulski (1977) found that earlier administration of hypnotics to hospitalized elderly patients resulted in more negative behavior (which is not necessarily bad) and an improvement in activities of daily living. Their conclusion was that time of administration should be in relation to normal sleep patterns. Gress and Bahr (1981), in a descriptive study of nocturnal behavior of 11 self-selected persons, aged 60 to 97, found that observation for three nights indicated a consistent individual pattern of sleep for each person, but that 2 A.M. was the time of greatest activity for the group as a whole.

Sleep patterns for the elderly may vary widely from the accepted efficient sleep of the young adult. Sleep apnea and the newer findings regarding use of hypnotics for the elderly offer challenging areas for nursing research.

Movement

In an experimental study, 30 nursing home residents were divided into a control and an experimental group; the investigators used movement therapy with the experimental group. Goldberg and Fitzpatrick (1980) found improvement in morale and in attitude toward aging and a trend toward greater self-esteem in the treated group.

Fitzpatrick and Donovan (1978) measured 60 persons aged 70 to 89, half of whom were institutionalized, for perception of time and for motor activity using the Motor Activity Rating Scale (MARS). The institutionalized were more oriented to the past than the noninstitutionalized group, a factor which seemed to be a function of institutionalization rather than of age. Patients in the institutionalized group had more gross body movements. The investigators questioned this finding as an artifact of their study, because the noninstitutionalized were not in their familiar setting and the institutionalized were. The MARS is an instrument that offers a method of measuring activity. Fitzpatrick and Donovan (1979), in a study of the reliability and validity of MARS, concluded that it was generally reliable and valid for assessing body position, body movements, and intensity of body movements. The interrater reliability varied from .97 on body position to .64 on moderate intensity; overall $r = .85$.

Important research questions to be studied include activity as a physiological need, as an important self-care action in depression, and to prevent confusional states. The question of activity versus rest in the elderly should be studied as should the phenomenon of restlessness.

Medication

Much of the nurse's time in long term care units is concerned with drug administration, observing the effect of multiple medications given to one patient, and meeting the regulatory mandates for updating medication orders by the physician. The Brown, Boosinger, Henderson, Rife, Rustea, Taylor, and Young survey (1977) of drug interaction showed that 100 out of 188 drug orders were high risk for drug interactions. Of 66 medication orders reviewed by physicians, 27 were potential drug-interactors. Lund (1979/1980) reported a descriptive study of decision-making and drug-management in two nursing homes based on questioning and observing of physicians, pharmacists, and nurses. The social organization of the nursing home and problems of the work place had precedence over bureaucratic regulation. Physicians relied on nurses' information and wrote drug orders to cover the nurses' decisions. The physician was not the decision maker envisioned in the legislated model but acted to support, interpret, and validate decisions already made by others, usually the nurse.

In a survey of drug-order updating in 109 nursing homes throughout the western states, Wolanin (1975) found that digitalis and tranquilizer orders were updated without physicians seeing the patient in 49.1 percent of the instances studied. Only 11 percent of the modification or discontinuance of the orders occurred on mailed forms, while 89 percent of the changes were associated with nurse-physician contact by telephone or discussion on the nursing unit of the patient's reaction to the medications.

In a three group experimental design, Kim and Grier (1981) studied nurses' instruction regarding medications to elderly clinic patients. They found that normally paced instructions (159 words per minute) given to one experimental group made no significant difference in understanding compared to the control group that received no instruction. The slow-paced instruction group (106 words per minute) differed significantly from the normal-paced group. Recognition was greater than recall, suggesting that written instruction should be given for reinforcement.

In long-term care units, drug administration requires nursing knowledge and clinical judgment in a situation where sharing of responsibility and having professional support are limited. The administration of p.r.n. medication (to be given if needed) and the multiple medications for one patient need extensive study by nurses. Pharmacokinetics of drugs in the elderly require knowledge of structural and functional changes that occur with aging in addition to knowledge of those that occur as a result of disease.

Relocation

Quayhagen (1977/1979) studied adaptation of the elderly to institutional relocation. She found that high environmental control, perceived well-being, low stress from personnel, low level of physical dependence, and low anxiety and depression were important predictors of adjustment in relocation. Two points of major stress in relocation lay between the first and second month and the second and third month.

Chenitz (1978/1979) found that the patient's initial adjustment and acceptance of the nursing home were factors in determining the stress of personnel. Patients who never adjusted were perceived as stressful by the nurses. In practice, communication barriers with patients who were confused or who suffered psychological problems were seen as stressful elements by physicians and nurses.

Grey (1978) used a patient profile to measure the physical and mental status of 137 elderly residents before they were moved and again 90 days after the move to determine change in status as a result of the move. The independent variable was a well organized plan and orientation for the move. The result was decreased mortality as compared to figures kept in prior years. There was improvement in locomotion, continence, motivation, and behavior in 59 of the residents. In a similar study of 14 elderly patients hospitalized over a long period of time and their move to a new long-term care unit, Wolanin (1978) found that careful planning and orientation resulted in no loss of mental status as measured by increased urinary incontinence, wandering, nocturnal wakefulness, and disorientation. Improvement in socialization, as demonstrated by interaction with other patients and staff, was found. There was no increase in mortality.

Dimond, King, and Burt (1979) studied 37 "well" persons between 42 and 99 with an average age of 66.5 years, some of whom were forced to move from one community to another and some who were not moved. This study indicated that coping resources could be used to identify those who were high risk for physical symptoms and depression as a result of moving. There was evidence that a sense of social isolation, presence or absence of a confidante, and living alone were important correlates of subjective well-being. Those with low coping skills were depressed and had more symptomatology nine months postmove.

Every admission to an acute care hospital or long-term care unit is a relocation to an environment over which nurses have a high degree of control. Research has pointed to some helpful interventions by nurses that prevent the frequently found change in mental status associated with relocation. There is abundant literature from other disciplines that can be applied to nursing and tested in the clinical situation.

Personal Space

Caregivers have felt the tension that arises when the elderly feel their personal space has been invaded or violated. Louis (1981) studied 40 people aged 65 to 90 on approach from the side and from the front. Elderly people require more space when approached from the side than from the front.

Beck (1978/1979) studied 60 elderly men and women and 60 college students using the Comfortable Interpersonal Distance (CID) scale (Duke & Navicki, 1972), which measures distance with the same and opposite sex. She found that the older the person, the greater the preferred distance; friends are preferred closer than strangers, and same sex persons are preferred closer than opposite sex persons. Beck saw interpersonal distance as an important variable in the area of communication.

Interpersonal space of the institutionalized elderly is an important concern for adjustment to relocation and should be studied. Research is needed for comfortable distance of nursing personnel and of location of personal possessions. None of the studies included use of sensory deficits as an intervening variable; the question of deafness and interpersonal space needs to be investigated.

Incontinence

Incontinence is a major concern of those who care for the elderly and indeed of the elderly themselves. Catanzaro (1981), in a qualitative study, exlored the meaning of incontinence with 126 individuals by gathering longitudinal and cross-sectional data through many forms of formal and informal interactions. Shame was the central property of a differentness perceived on the basis of urinary bladder dysfunction. In a descriptive study of 65 patients with cardiovascular accident (first stroke), Adams (1966) found an 83 percent incidence of incontinence. It was associated with age, inability to walk, speech pathology, dependence on others for care, and an inability to perform simple commands. It was also associated with hemiplegia with loss of proprioception.

Behavior modification or operant conditioning was the independent variable in two studies of controlling incontinence in elderly men. Carpenter and Simon (1960) used a two-hour habit training, with rewards for success and disapproval as punishment for failure. Wearing personal clothing was the best reward and wearing hospital or different clothing was the greatest punishment. Investigators assumed that incontinence was always a behavior problem, and no tests were made for other causes of incontinence. Grosicki (1968) studied 18 elderly men over age 63 for 12 weeks. Social reinforcement was given when they were dry, and later this was changed to tokens, which could be used as money, if the patients used a commode voluntarily. There was no difference in the incidence of incontinence as compared to a control group without rewards. Again, the problem of organic dysfunction was not taken into account.

The studies cited above, with the exception of Catanzaro (1981) are at least 14 years old and have not been followed by published work although this is a major problem in long term care. Adams's (1966) descriptive study should be followed with more research of elderly patients with orthopedic surgery and of the wheel chair bound.

Family Caregivers

Four studies of caregivers offer a background for understanding the nurse in this role. Mack (1952) reported the adjustment of chronically ill old people under home care in the first issue of *Nursing Research*. She found a relationship between favorable family attitudes and good adjustment by the patient to chronic illness. Compared to "normal" old people, those with chronic illness tended to be less happy, less active, and less well adjusted. In a qualitative field study, Archbold (1980/1981) analyzed the results of intensive observation of 30 Caucasian women who cared for an aging parent. Two caregiving roles were identified: the provider who supplied direct care, and the care manager who found and managed the resources for care. The provider suffered loss of freedom and privacy and knew daily irritation and guilt. The manager had time limitations, fatigue, financial drain, and guilt.

A descriptive study of 74 family relationships in which a caregiver and frail elderly homebound patient were observed and interviewed led to identification of two groups, 44 with good relationships and 30 with abusive relationships (Phillips, 1980/1981). The two groups differed on social supports, expectations of the caregivers, and perceptions of the caregivers. Motives, attitudes, family structure, and nature of the family relationships all contributed to the differences between a good and an abusive relationship. The nurse's role for intervention in such cases is not as clear as it is in child abuse, for the caregiver is often an elderly spouse. Hirschfeld (1978/1979), in a study of 30 families living with an elderly person who had senile brain disease, found that the lower the tension, the greater the quality of the dyadic relationship and management ability and the need for institutionalization on the basis of family exhaustion. She concluded that there was a need for programs to alleviate the impact on the family, and she recommended that nurses develop knowledge and skills to measure family impact and ability to cope with impairment.

The moral and political climate tends toward more home care and less institutionalization for the elderly. More research by nurses will be required if they are to understand the caregiver in the home and the dynamics of caring for the elderly person, whether by the aging spouse or by the adult children who may be encountering their own aging process. For this research, there are definitional, political, and methodological issues that will confront the investigator.

Support and Stress

Fuller and Larson (1980) investigated the relationship between stressful life changes and health among 50 persons aged 51 to 89. Stress-producing life events correlated negatively with functional health, and there was no evidence that emotional support modified the effects of life events on functional health. On the other hand, Dimond (1981) found that supportive networks, successful past coping skills, and a lack of concurrent losses were important to adaptation to grief after the death of a spouse.

The research cited above confirms the need for additional studies of the bereaved elderly. The need for longitudinal studies, identified by Dimond (1981), is also true for many other concerns investigated by nurses.

Changes in Mental Status

Using the grounded theory approach of Glaser and Strauss (1967), Wolanin (1976) studied 30 confused elderly in a nursing home, using participant observation, interviews with staff, and clinical records. The purpose was to determine what behaviors of the elderly led to the label of confusion by the staff. Two kinds of behavior were identified: those that made the patient socially inaccessible and those that made him cognitively inaccessible. Characteristics of the confused elderly included sensoriperceptual problems, hypotension, decreased mobility, and multiple medications, with digitalis derivatives, tranquilizers, and diuretics most common. Confusional states varied widely from individual to individual.

In a descriptive study of 91 elderly who were admitted for repair of hip fracture, Williams, Holloway, Winn, Wolanin, Lawler, Westwick, and Chin (1979) found that admission and preoperative confusional states were best indicators of postoperative confusion when observed on the first, third, and fifth postoperative days (POD). On the first POD, the 33 percent incidence of confusion, according to the instruments designed by the investigators, was confirmed by staff and personal report by patients who recognized change in their mental status. Problems with urinary elimination, deafness, and immobility contributed to continuing confusional states on the fifth POD. Nursing interventions to relieve confusional states varied from none to those that comforted, relieved pain, or removed mucus plugs. Patients did not recognize that nurses offered any intervention.

Chisholm, Deniston, Igrisan, and Barbus (1982) investigated all patients age 60 or over who were admitted to a hospital for any cause. Among the 99 patients, they found a 55 percent incidence of acute confusion as measured by a tool designed for the study. Only 5 percent had been labeled confused on admission. Average time of onset of the confusional state was 6 ½ days postadmission, with a range of 1 to 26 days. Two instruments were given with the reported study, one for assessment of confusion, and one for determining the cause for the confusion. They have face validity; reliability was not stated.

Roslaniec and Fitzpatrick (1979) tested mental status change in the elderly hospitalized on admission and on Day 4. Using an investigator constructed instrument, which was assessed for reliability and validity, they found no significant difference in attention, ability to calculate, or to concentrate but significant deterioration in consciousness, orientation, abstract reasoning, and impairment of ability to do memory tasks on Day 4. The independent variable was four days in the hospital.

With personal control as a conceptual framework, Hill (1982) used behavioral instruction (i.e., rehearsal of ways to reduce discomfort, get out of bed, and practice self-care skills) with patients who were to have sensory alteration surgery. The dependent variables were degree of anxiety and depression, ability to ambulate, hospital days, postoperative confusional states, orientation, and the first time ventured away from home postoperatively. Using four groups of ten each, Hill's design included a control group, one experimental group with behavioral rehearsal, a second with a sensory information tape, and a third using both the sensory information tape and behavioral rehearsal. Sensory information reduced anxiety and depression and shortened the time before venturing away from home. The group that was given the combined treatment ventured from home first. It was found that 17.5 percent of the patients had indeterminate stimulus events such as visual, auditory, body touch, or combined experiences, usually in the late afternoon or early evening. There were no significant differences in confusion and orientation among the groups.

Twenty depressed elderly people in a psychiatric hospital were interviewed to determine needs for specific nursing interventions (Dominick, 1968). Interpersonal actions, satisfaction of need for knowledge, and satisfaction of social needs were the interventions cited as needed and in that order.

In research of elderly patients with hip fracture, Carlson (1968) found that they showed earlier responsibility for their own recovery and rehabilitation when offered sensory stimulation including auditory, visual, olfactory, and tactile stimuli. In an experimental study involving touch as the independent variable, Langland and Panicucci (1982) found a significant increase in verbal response when measured by the Pfeiffer (1975) Short Portable Mental Status Questionnaire (SPMSQ). Touch on the forearm conveyed relational aspects of communication.

The introduction of a puppy changed the behavior of elderly men as measured by smiles, verbalization, open eyes, and leaning toward the stimulus (Robb, Boyd, & Pristash, 1980). A wine bottle and a plant did not elicit the same degree of response.

Using an experimental design to test the efficacy of reality orientation, Hogstel (1979) placed calendars on the wall and used clocks and a one-to-one event daily for her experimental group. She also offered them five 30-minute classes of reality orientation weekly for three weeks. There was no measurable difference between the control and the experimental group, but less apathy was noted in the experimental group.

Also using an experimental design, Dennis (1976) included three groups to investigate the use of resocialization therapy to decrease depression and increase life satisfaction in the elderly. The control group had no treatment, the first experimental group received special attention, and the second experimental group was given resocialization therapy for 12 weeks. There was a significant difference as measured on the Zung (1970) self-administered depression scale and a decrease in life satisfaction in the remotivation group. The conclusion was that the remotivation group realized they had no control over their lives.

Elderly people were divided into three groups on the basis of mental status by Gray and Stevenson (1980). Resocialization therapy was offered to each group in weekly sessions for four months. All groups showed improvement, but the most confused group showed the greatest improvement.

Voelkel (1978) found resocialization therapy more effective than reality orientation. Twenty persons age 80 to 95 were placed randomly in two groups on the basis of testing with the SPMSQ (Pfeiffer, 1975). One group received reality orientation and the other resocialization therapy three times weekly for six weeks. The results indicated that the resocialization group showed greater improvement than the reality orientation group. However, two persons who had hearing problems did not improve their mental status score, indicating that group therapy is not the best means of therapy for hearing-impaired persons. The research report is exceptional in its candid discussion of the conditions of research with the elderly in nursing homes.

The numerous small studies of nurse intervention using group therapy point to the possibility of using a well designed study with a network of investigators to develop a large sample that could be studied in relation to age, mental status, health, time in institution, depression, and the nursing intervention. The role of health or physiological causes in the confusional states has not been considered in depth. Nursing interventions for depression in the elderly have had almost no study.

LeSage (1979/1980) reported an initial attempt to use color vision as an indicator of digoxin toxicity. This noninvasive test could be used by nurses in long term care units and in homes where laboratory tests are not available. LeSage is continuing this research, which could lead to a development of noninvasive tests for other body deficiencies. Such tests would allow nurses to validate their clinical observations quickly and take remedial action in the early stages.

PROBLEMS IN CONDUCTING CLINICAL GERIATRIC NURSING RESEARCH

Conceptual Issues

The first conceptual issue that should be dealt with in any study of the aged is the inexact definition of aging. The chronological definition which uses the Social Security turning point of 65 establishes a floor. Unfortunately, this is not maintained throughout research or policy decisions based on research. Various people define aging as beginning at 60 or at 55 in some cases where a larger statistic is desired. With the increase in longevity, the term "aged" may include the very young and vigorous 60-year-old with a centenarian who is 40 years older and two generations apart. There is little homogeneity among cohorts of the aged and none in samples that include ranges covering 20 to 30 years of life. Such differences in definition preclude any comparison of one study with another because of the age groups included.

Chronological age is often the only criterion used in selection of a sample. Health of the older individual may be more crucial than the chronological age in developing a homogeneous sample, and sensoriperceptual deficits can create another variable that must be considered with age itself.

The second issue to be confronted in research on aging is who represents the aged. Studies are usually done on a sample that is convenient to the researcher. Congregate-living or institutionalized elderly, who represent 5 to 10 percent of the total population over the age of 65, are studied at the expense of the 90 to 95 percent whom it would require greater effort to reach. Very few studies are done of the aged in acute care settings, yet the elderly occupy 35 to 50 percent of the beds in acute care. Elderly persons in long term care were not overstudied; the older person in the home or in the acute care setting was studied even less frequently.

The ethics of studying the elderly has become a concern of some researchers (Archbold, 1981; Cogliano, 1979; Davis, 1981; Wolanin,

1980). The need for informed consent has unclear implications for the older person who may have impaired sensory or cognitive ability. Yet these people need to be studied as one of the most vulnerable groups of aging who need nursing care. All of these issues include grave questions of the means and ends of research, of the individual good and the common good, and of the whole overlaid by legal rights.

Finally, conceptual concerns themselves are issues. Are the right questions being asked and studied, or are the easy questions being investigated? Are nurse researchers investigating the concerns that have high priority for the practitioner? Do the conceptual concerns studied lead to abstraction and theory that will assist the practitioner? Wald and Leonard (1964) suggested that what has been overlooked is a need to begin from practical nursing experience and develop concepts from an analysis of the clinical experience rather than try to make borrowed concepts fit. In their Delphi study to identify research priorities for long term care in gerontological nursing, Brower and Christ (Note 2) found the first five in the order given:

1. study the prevention, formation, and treatment of decubiti;
2. describe coping mechanisms needed by family and patient after discharge;
3. find ways to increase physician interest in geriatrics;
4. determine age differences in relation to medications;
5. determine methods of improving gerontological preparation of nursing students and ancillary and nursing staff.

Methodological Concerns

Gunter and Miller (1977) wrote of the need for longitudinal instead of cross-sectional studies that have been used in the interest of saving time. The need remains, for nurse researchers still work under constraint of time, and very few nursing research projects are funded; therefore methods that produce results rather quickly have been chosen. Longitudinal studies suffer attrition of sample, especially with the older population. But longitudinal studies that are being conducted at The Duke University Geriatric Center are the studies that offer the best information about aging over time. No two cohorts have had the same life experience; in fact, no cohort is homogeneous in any respect except for the fact of birthdate.

The use of the questionnaire as a means of collecting data has its limitations for the elderly, whose life experience makes almost any question ambiguous. Poor vision and lack of reading skills make a questionnaire of limited value for representing information about the elderly population. Statistical analysis of answer sheets may be an analysis of the older person's confusion with the answer sheet method. Interviews with the elderly have their problems; the interviewer may be an intervening variable.

The problem of sampling, mentioned under conceptual issues, is one of the grave issues that the person designing a study must face. Who is represented? Do the ill elderly speak for all elderly because they are accessible while their cohorts may be playing golf or running marathons? Is the sample appropriate for the research design, or does it serve the disparate needs of the researcher only? Is the problem one which is related to social problems of mankind in general, or is it a problem of aging? Is the question one that can be studied by other disciplines, or is it a nursing question for which no other discipline has the concepts, methods, and tools for study?

The problems in geriatric clinical nursing are still relatively unstudied. We do not know the important dependent variables. Grounded theory methodology (Glaser & Strauss, 1967) could well serve as the technique to identify those variables.

Some phenomena are not found in one location in sufficient quantity to afford a sample of the size recommended for statistical analysis. Does this mean that this particular problem should not be studied, or does it mean that a new methodology and statistical analysis are required in clinical geriatric research? Statistical methods have been inherited from other disciplines where the problems are totally different. Fruitflies offer fewer complications than human beings full of years.

Methodology is often a matter of compromises: what begins as ideal must be changed to meet reality. Hinshaw (1981) said that individuals conducting clinical research must face the type of investigations that nurses undertake, i.e., projects that involve human subjects in a field setting over which they have limited control. Clinical research usually involves a series of compromises during the course of investigation.

Need for More Descriptive Studies

Although there are many descriptive studies, there is still a need for observing, counting, and describing as the first level of factor isolation and factor relating (Dickoff & James, 1968). The second level, depiction of whole situations, requires taking tremendous amounts of data into consideration when dealing with the elderly. The need to show cause and effect has often resulted in suspending efforts to develop the first two levels, which must be adequate to lay a foundation for experimental studies.

Instrument Construction

There are few instruments to use in clinical geriatric nursing research. Borrowing tools from other disciplines has not given nurse researchers instruments for collecting data in clinical research. Borrowed tools are tempting, but they do not answer nursing questions, and they result in research *by* nurses but often not *about* nursing. Courses in instrumentation will undoubtedly help to close the gap, but at this time clinical nurse researchers must fashion their own tools. This means the delay of research while the proper instrument is designed, tested, and standardized (Ventura, Hinshaw, & Atwood, 1981).

Often the experimenter assumes that causation works in one direction or that independent variables are causes and dependent variables show effect. In exchanges between two human beings, especially in the nurse-patient interaction, the arrows of causation point in both directions (Tyler, 1981). For the instrument designer, this presents a tremendous challenge.

Analysis of Data

Quantitative analysis leads to quick and easy answers by computerization. Vast amounts of data can be handled, and interpretation of findings is simplified. Statistical methods frequently focus on inference and confirmatory analysis, in contrast to description and exploratory analysis. However, information about things that cannot be quantified but that are forced into scales as if they can be, has resulted in not examining the data for trends and serendipitous findings (Jacobsen, 1981). Careful perusal of data obtained in studies with the elderly is still the analytical method of choice at this stage of clinical nursing research. It is still necessary to count, describe, and categorize. The computer will assist in counting and point to associations, but it does not have insight, it does not define categories that arise from clinical experience. There is still a need for the plodding efforts and insights of the dedicated researcher.

SUMMARY

Accessibility and retrieval of the research findings are the responsiblity of the investigator at this time. The investigator must compete with other researchers for precious space in journals that report research. This report has used Medline searches, journals, and doctoral dissertations to glean published and accessible research reports. The paucity of clinical research that is available may be judged by the fact that this review represents published research from 1952 to 1982.

A clinical nursing research digest would enhance the clinician's chances of learning about relevant research in the field of nursing the aged. A special journal to report research in nursing care of the aged is not unrealistic.

REFERENCE NOTES

1. MacRae, I. *Priorities for clinical nursing research in gerontology.* Paper presented at the Scientific Sessions, Gerontological Society of America, Toronto, Canada, November 1981.
2. Brower, H. T., & Christ, M. A. Personal communication, 1982.

REFERENCES

Adams, M. Urinary incontinence in the acute phase of cerebral vascular accident. *Nursing Research,* 1966, *15,* 100–108.

Ankenbrandt, M. A., & Tanner, L. K. Role-delineated and informal nurse-teaching and food selection behavior of geriatric patients. *Nursing Research,* 1971, *20,* 61–64.

Archbold, P. G. Impact of parent-caring on women. (Doctoral dissertation, University of California, San Francisco, 1980.) *Dissertation Abstracts International,* 1981, *41,* 2967B-2968B. (University Microfilms No. 8104158)

Archbold, P. G. Ethical issues in selection of a theoretical framework for gerontological nursing research. *Journal of Gerontological Nursing,* 1981, *7,* 408–416.

Baekeland, F., & Hartmann, E. Reported sleep characteristics: Effects of age, sleep length, and psychiatric impairment. *Comparative Psychiatry,* 1971, *12,* 141–147.

Baltes, M. M., & Zerbe, M. B. Reestablishing self-feeding in a nursing home resident. *Nursing Research,* 1976, *25,* 24–26.

Basson, P. H. The gerontological nursing literature search: Study and results. *Nursing Research,* 1967, *16,* 267–272.

Beck, C. M. The comfortable interpersonal distance of the aged. (Doctoral dissertation, Texas Women's University, 1978.) *Dissertation Abstracts International,* 1979, *39,* 1208B. (University Microfilms No. 7815586)

Brimmer, P. The past, present and future in gerontological nursing research. *Journal of Gerontological Nursing,* 1979, *5*(1), 27–34.

Brown, M. I., Basson, P. H., & Burchett, D. E. *Nursing care of the aged.* (U.S. Public Health Service Publication No. 1603,) Washington, D.C.: U.S. Government Printing Office, 1967.

Brown, M. M., Boosinger, J. K., Henderson, M., Rife, S. S., Rustea, J. K., Taylor, O., & Young, W. W. Drug interaction. *Nursing Research,* 1977, *26,* 47–52.

Carlson, S. Selected sensory input and life satisfaction of immobilized geriatric female patients. In American Nurses Association, *ANA clinical sessions.* New York: Appleton-Century-Crofts, 1968.

Carpenter, H., & Simon, R. The effect of several methods of training on long term incontinent patients. *Nursing Research,* 1960, *9,* 17–22.

Catanzaro, M. "Shamefully different": A personal meaning of urinary bladder dysfunction. In M. Batey, (Ed.), *Communicating nursing research* (Vol. 14). Boulder, Colo.: Western Interstate Commission for Higher Education, 1981.

Chenitz, C. Acceptance of the *Standards of Geriatric Nursing Practice* and perceptions of satisfying and stressful elements in practice by geriatric nurses. (Doctoral dissertation, Columbia University Teachers College, 1978.) *Dissertation Abstracts International,* 1979, *39,* 4810B–4811B. (University Microfilms No. 7908986)

Chisholm, S. E., Deniston, O. L., Igrisan, R. M., & Barbus, A. J. Prevalence of confusion in elderly hospitalized patients. *Journal of Gerontological Nursing,* 1982, *8,* 87–90.

Cogliano, J. F. Clinical research in the nursing home: One viewpoint. *Journal of Gerontological Nursing,* 1979, *5*(6), 39–43.

Davis, A. Ethical considerations in gerontological nursing research. *Geriatric Nursing,* 1981, *2,* 269–272.

Dennis, H. Remotivation therapy for the elderly: A surprising outcome. *Journal of Gerontological Nursing,* 1976, *2*(6), 28–30.

DeWalt, E. Effect of timed hygienic measures on oral mucosa in a group of elderly patients. *Nursing Research,* 1975, *24,* 104–108.

Dickoff, J., & James, P. Theory of theories: A position paper. *Nursing Research,* 1968, *17,* 197–203.

Dimond, M. Bereavement and the elderly: A critical review with implications for nursing. *Journal of Advanced Nursing,* 1981, *6,* 461–470.

Dimond, M., King, K., & Burt, M. Forced relocation and the elderly: Identifying facilitators and barriers to adjustment. *Selected papers from the Clinical and Scientific Sessions.* Kansas City, Mo.: American Nurses Association, 1979.

Dittmar, S. S., & Dulski, T. Early administration of sleep medication to the hospitalized elderly. *Nursing Research,* 1977, *26,* 299–293.

Dominick, J. R. Nursing care factors in psychotic depressive reactions in elderly patients. *Perspectives in Psychiatric Care*, 1968, *6*, 28–32.

Duke, M., & Navicki, S. A new measure in social learning model for interpersonal distance. *Journal of Experimental Research in Personality*, 1972, *6*, 119–132.

Fitzpatrick, J. J., & Donovan, M. J. Temporal experience and motor behavior among the aged. *Research in Nursing and Health*, 1978, *1*, 60–68.

Fitzpatrick, J. J., & Donovan, M. J. A follow-up study of the reliability and validity of the Motor Activity Rating Scale. *Nursing Research*, 1979, *28*, 179–181.

Fuller, S. S., & Larson, S. B. Life events, emotional support and health of older people. *Research in Nursing and Health*, 1980, *3*, 81–89.

Gerber, R. M., & Van Ort, S. R. Topical application of insulin in decubitus ulcers. *Nursing Research*, 1979, *28*, 16–19.

Glaser, B. G., & Strauss, A. L. *The discovery of grounded theory*. Chicago: Aldine, 1967.

Goldberg, W. G., & Fitzpatrick, J. J. Movement therapy with the aged. *Nursing Research*, 1980, *29*, 339–346.

Gray, P., & Stevenson, J. C. Changes in verbal interaction among members of resocialization groups. *Journal of Gerontological Nursing*, 1980, *6*, 86–90.

Gress, L. D., & Bahr, R. T. Nocturnal behavior of selected institutionalized adults. *Journal of Gerontological Nursing*, 1981, *7*, 86–98.

Grey, C. Moving 137 elderly residents to a new facility. *Journal of Gerontological Nursing*, 1978, *4*(6), 34–38.

Grosicki, J. P. Effective operant conditioning modification of incontinence in neuropsychiatric geriatric patients. *Nursing Research*, 1968, *17*, 302–311.

Gunter, L., & Miller, J. Toward a nursing gerontology. *Nursing Research*, 1977, *26*, 208–221.

Hayter, J., & McPhetridge, L. M. Study of decubitus care. *Journal of Gerontological Nursing*, 1976, *2*(3), 24–27.

Hill, B. J. Sensory information, behavioral instructions and coping with sensory alteration surgery. *Nursing Research*, 1982, *31*, 17–21.

Hinshaw, A. S. Problems in doing research—Compromise? Always! Where? How much? *Western Journal of Nursing Research*, 1981, *3*, 109–111.

Hirschfeld, M. J. Families living with senile brain disease (Doctoral dissertation, University of California, San Francisco, 1978). *Dissertation Abstracts International*, 1979, *39*, 3241B–3242B. (University Microfilms No. 7900838)

Hogstel, M. O. Use of reality orientation with aged confused patients. *Nursing Research*, 1979, *28*, 161–165.

Jacobsen, B. S. Know thy data. *Nursing Research*, 1981, *30*, 254–255.

Kayser-Jones, J. S. Gerontological nursing research revisited. *Journal of Gerontological Nursing*, 1981, *7*, 217–221.

Kim, K. K., & Grier, M. R. Pacing effects of medication instruction for the elderly. *Journal of Gerontological Nursing*, 1981, *7*, 464–468.

King, P. A. Foot assessment of the elderly. *Journal of Gerontological Nursing*, 1978, *4*(6), 47–52.

Lamb, K. Effect of positioning of post-operative fractured hip patients as related to comfort. *Nursing Research*, 1979, *28*, 291–293.

Langland, R. M., & Panicucci, C. L. Effects of touch on communication with elderly confused patients. *Journal of Gerontological Nursing*, 1982, *8*, 152–155.

LeSage, J. M. Acquired color vision deficiency in people taking digoxin (Doctoral dissertation, Texas Women's University, 1979). *Dissertation Abstracts International*, 1980, *40*, 5608B–5609B. (University Microfilms No. 8012171)

Lewis, H. E., & Masterson, J. P. Sleep and wakefulness in the Artic. *Lancet*, 1957, *1*, 1262–1266.

Louis, M. Personal space boundary needs of elderly persons: An empirical study. *Journal of Gerontological Nursing*, 1981, *7*, 395–400.

Lund, M. D. E. The social organization of drug management in two nursing homes (Doctoral dissertation, University of Illinois at the Medical Center, 1979). *Dissertation Abstracts International*, 1980, *40*, 1632B. (University Microfilms No. 7922895)

Mack, M. J. The personal adjustment of chronically ill old people under home care. *Nursing Research*, 1952, *1*(1), 9–30.

Managan, D. Older adults: A community survey of health needs. *Nursing Research*, 1974, *23*, 426–432.

Neely, E., & Patrick, M. L. Problems of aged persons taking medications at home. *Nursing Research*, 1968, *17*, 52–55.

Pacini, C. M., & Fitzpatrick, J. J. Sleep pattern of hospitalized and non-hospitalized aged individuals. *Journal of Gerontological Nursing*, 1982, *8*, 332–337.

Pfeiffer, E. A. A short portable mental status questionnaire for the assessment of organic brain deficit in elderly patients. *Journal of American Geriatric Society*, 1975, *23*, 433–441.

Phillips, L. R. F. Family relationships between two samples of frail elderly individuals (Doctoral dissertation, University of Arizona, 1980). *Dissertation Abstracts International*, 1981, *41*, 3741B. (University Microfilms No. 8106934)

Quayhagen, M. P. Adaptation of elderly to institutional relocation: A conceptual model (Doctoral dissertation, University of California, San Francisco, 1977). *Dissertation Abstracts International*, 1979, *39*, 4817B. (University Microfilms No. 7900842)

Robb, S. S., Boyd, M., & Pristash, C. L. A wine bottle, plant and puppy: Catalysts for social behavior. *Journal of Gerontological Nursing*, 1980, *6*, 721–728.

Roslaniec, A., & Fitzpatrick, J. J. Changes in mental status of older adults with 4 days hospitalization. *Research in Nursing and Health*, 1979, *2*, 177–187.

Schank, M. J. A survey of well elderly: Their foot problems, practices and needs. *Journal of Gerontological Nursing*, 1977, *3*(6), 10–15.

Steadman, P. E., Schenk, E. A., & Walker, S. K. Reducing devices for pressure sores with respect to nursing care procedures. *Nursing Research*, 1980, *29*, 228–230.

Stotsky, E. A., & Rhetts, J. E. Changing attitudes toward the mentally ill in nursing homes. *Nursing Research*, 1966, *15*, 175–177.

Tyler, L. E. More stately mansions—Psychology extends its boundaries. *Annual Review of Psychology*, 1981, *32*, 1–20.

Van Drimmelen, J., & Rollins, H. F. Evaluation of a commonly used oral hygienic agent. *Nursing Research*, 1969, *18*, 327–332.

Ventura, M. R., Hinshaw, A. S., & Atwood, J. Instrumentation: The next step. *Nursing Research,* 1981, *30,* 257.
Verhonick, P. J. Decubitus ulcer observations measured objectively. *Nursing Research,* 1961, *10,* 211–214.
Voelkel, D. A study of reality orientation and socialization of confused elderly. *Journal of Gerontological Nursing,* 1978, *4*(3), 13–18.
Wald, F. S., & Leonard, R. C. Toward development of nursing practice theory. *Nursing Research,* 1964, *13,* 310.
Williams, M., Holloway, J., Winn, J., Wolanin, M. O., Lawler, M. L., Westwick, C. R., & Chin, M. H. Nursing activities and acute confusional states in elderly hip fractured patients. *Nursing Research,* 1979, *28,* 25–35.
Wolanin, M. O. Process criterion vs. impact criterion to measure quality of care in nursing homes. In T. Talbot (Ed.), *Proceedings of First North American Symposium on Long Term Care Administration.* Washington, D.C.: American College of Nursing Home Administration, 1975.
Wolanin, M. O. Confusion study: Grounded theory as methodology. In M. Batey (Ed.), *Communicating nursing research* (Vol. 7). Boulder, Colo.: Western Interstate Commission on Higher Education, 1976.
Wolanin, M. O. Relocation of the elderly. *Journal of Gerontolgcial Nursing,* 1978, *4*(3), 47–51.
Wolanin, M. O. Research and the aged. In A. M. Davis & J. D. Krueger (Eds.), *Patients, nurses and ethics.* New York: American Journal of Nursing, 1980.
Zung, W. W. Mood disturbances in the elderly. *Gerontologist,* 1970, *10,* 2–4.

CHAPTER 5

Nursing Research on Death, Dying, and Terminal Illness: Development, Present State, and Prospects

JEANNE QUINT BENOLIEL
COMMUNITY HEALTH CARE SYSTEMS DEPARTMENT
UNIVERSITY OF WASHINGTON

CONTENTS

OVERVIEW OF DEATH-RELATED RESEARCH

Presented in this review is an historical overview on the development of death research in general followed by an analysis of nursing research in death, dying, and terminal illness. Of necessity, some death-related areas

The bibliographic material on which this review is based was collected with the assistance of Training Grant 1 D23 NU00210–01 from the Division of Nursing, Health Resources Administration, Department of Health and Human Services. Considerable help in locating and sorting materials was provided by Linda K. Birenbaum, Fotini L. Georgiadou, Barbara B. Germino, and Christina M. Mumma. Appreciation is due to Lesley F. Degner, Helen P. Glass, Christina M. Gow, Sherry Johnson-Soderberg, Sylvia Drake Paige, Geraldine V. Padilla, Catherine M. Saunders, and Mary L. S. Vachon for providing copies of published and unpublished materials for use in this review. The organization of the report was suggested to me by a review written by Gunther Luschen in the *Annual Review of Sociology* (Vol. 6), 1980.

of interest to nurses were not included. Among these topics are suicide and abortion, each of which deserves consideration in its own right. Owing to difficulties in accessibility, only occasionally is research included that was conducted outside the North American continent.

The methods used for information retrieval precede a discussion of the origins of death research in nursing, some observations on methodology, and an analysis of substantive contributions to the field. In the review, questions are raised about the present state of knowledge relevant to terminal illness and care, the contribution of death research to the discipline at large, and some practical implications for nursing as a profession.

Historically, human death and dying as subjects for scientific investigation are phenomena of the 20th century. Their rapid emergence following World War II can be tied to the rapid expansion of organized science, the mental health movement's interest in death, a depersonalization of many human experiences associated with technologic development, and a pervasive death anxiety coming in the aftermath of Hiroshima (Benoliel, 1978). Prior to 1940, pioneer contributions to this domain of knowledge came from anthropological investigations of death customs in primitive societies (Bendann, 1930; Benedict, 1934; Frazier, 1913–1922; Kroeber, 1927) and from psychoanalytic perspectives on the meaning of death. Freud's concepts of unconscious immortality (1915) and the "death instinct" (1920) were central to the latter development. In sociology, Eliot (1930) noted the paucity of research about family responses to grief and identified the need for a social psychology of bereavement (1933). Among the first to write about philosophic and practical matters affecting the care of the dying was Worcester (1935).

The beginnings of death-related research in psychiatry, sociology, and psychology came between 1940 and 1960. Anthony's (1940) classic study of children's awareness of death paved the way for Lindemann's (1944) empirical analysis of acute grief processes and Eissler's (1955) seminal work on psychiatric relationships with the dying patient. An essay by anthropologist Gorer (1956) argued persuasively that death had replaced sex as an object of prudery and avoidance in modern society, and his ideas influenced the thinking of many western scholars. In sociology, Habenstein and Lamers (1955) investigated the role of the funeral director as it evolved in the United States and later did a cross-cultural analysis of burial and funeral customs throughout the world (1960). Marris (1958) studied the bereavement reactions of widows in London, and Volkart and Michael (1957) proposed that bereavement practices were related directly to variations in cultural values and kinship structures. Feifel (1959) began his pioneer work on attitudes toward death and, equally important, edited a collection of essays that emphasized multidisciplinary inquiry into the meaning of death and legitimized empirical research in the field.

After 1960 interest in the study of death spread across a variety of academic and applied fields. Between 1960 and 1970, significant contributions to knowledge about the personal, interpersonal, and social meanings of death and dying came from investigations by Fulton (1961), Kalish (1963), Gorer (1965), Glaser and Strauss (1965, 1968), Hinton (1967), Sudnow (1967), and Kübler-Ross (1969). Important theoretical formulations and conceptual perspectives came out of Bowlby's (1960) work on grief and mourning in childhood, Weisman and Hackett's (1961) thinking on dying and predilection to death, Blauner's (1966) analysis of social structure and death, and Lifton's (1968) study of the impact and aftermath of exposure to mass death. In philosophy, Choron (1963) traced the development of western ideas about death, and Koestenbaum (1964) analyzed the different meanings of death of the self and death of another. The multidisciplinary nature of death inquiry was shown again in collections of essays by Fulton (1965) and Toynbee, Mant, Smart, Hinton, Yudkin, Rhode, Heywood, and Price (1968) and in the creation of the Foundation of Thanatology (1968). Saunders (1969) described how her work in hospice care began out of concern with the clinical problem of intractable pain. In 1966 Kalish and Kastenbaum (Note 1) initiated a newsletter that served as the forerunner for *Omega: The Journal on Death and Dying*. (The journal was published initially in 1970.) These and other early efforts provided theoretical and empirical foundations for a proliferation of research and clinical study on death, dying, bereavement, and terminal illness in the decade that followed.

INFORMATION RETRIEVAL AND ANALYSIS

The search for nursing research in death, dying, and terminal illness was done in several ways. A Medline search of health-sciences literature was performed for the years 1969 through 1981, producing a total of 864 citations. The list was perused to identify publications likely to be research reports, and copies of articles deemed appropriate for the review were obtained. *Indexes of Dissertation Abstracts International* for the years 1965 through 1981 were examined to locate death-related studies by nurses and about nurses and death by other investigators. Location of doctoral disserta-tions on death and dying for the 1970s was aided by a published list by Santora (1980a, 1980b). All issues of known journals identified with inquiry into death-related matters were reviewed for relevant research reports. These journals were *Omega, Life-Threatening Behavior* (changed to *Suicide and Life-Threatening Behavior* in 1975), *Essence,* and *Death Education.* All issues of *Nursing Research* were reviewed for appropriate research reports; the abstracts published in that journal between 1960 and 1978 provided helpful leads to other relevant publications. Other nursing journals reviewed were *Research in Nursing and Health, Advances in Nursing Science, Cancer Nursing, Oncology Nursing Forum,* and *Western Journal of Nursing Research.* Also searched were volumes 1 through 15 of *Communicating Nursing Research* published by the Western Interstate Commission for Higher Education beginning in 1968. Copies of published and unpublished papers, articles, and reports were obtained through corre-spondence with known nurse-investigators in the field.

Five criteria were developed for use in evaluating both published and unpublished papers and reports. These criteria were: (a) the inclusion of a theoretical or conceptual framework; (b) a clear statement of methodology including consideration of design, sample, instruments, and analytic pro-cedures; (c) a discussion of validity and reliability; (d) methods of analysis appropriate to the data; and (e) a logical and conservative interpretation of the findings. The guidelines were applied in modified form to papers dealing primarily with conceptual issues.

EMERGENCE OF DEATH RESEARCH IN NURSING

Death-related research in nursing began to appear during the 1960s. Prior to that time, the nursing literature on death and dying was meager and focused principally on the technical tasks to be done at and around the time of death (Quint, 1967). An exception was Norris's (1955) article on the psycho-logical stresses and tensions for nurses in caring for dying patients and their families. Peplau's (1952) ideas on the central importance of interpersonal relations in nursing stimulated the thinking of many nurses, and this influence was reflected in several publications emphasizing the nurse's responsibility for offering emotional support in long-term care (Blumberg & Drummond, 1963), when the prognosis was negative (Ujhely, 1963), and following a stillbirth (Bruce, 1962). Reports of clinical studies in the

1960s resulted from nurses' questions about ways of helping patients adjust to inoperable cancer (Kyle, 1964), different forms of pain experienced by patients (Mieding, 1964) and actions by nurses in the administration of analgesics (Buckeridge, Geiser, & Thomas, 1964). These areas of clinical concern subsequently became subjects for systematic nursing inquiry.

Formal nursing research into death, dying, and terminal illness began in the decade between 1960 and 1970. Its character was greatly influenced by the movement of nurses into other disciplines for doctoral study. This diversity in educational background brought to nursing research in death and dying three kinds of variability: orientation toward the meaning of research, theoretical frameworks within which to study identified problems, and methodologies used for scientific investigations. Not surprisingly, studies by nurses reflected the influence of these ties to other disciplines. The fields of education, sociology, and psychology played a major part in the development of nursing research on death and dying.

Forty-nine dissertations dealing with death-related questions of interest to nursing were found for the years 1963 through 1981. To identify nurse-investigators whose work was in fields other than nursing, the names of investigators were cross-checked with the *Directory of Nurses with Doctoral Degrees* (1980). It is conceivable that some nurse-investigators were not identified either because they were not listed or because the titles of their dissertations did not include words used in the search. The 15 studies by nonnurse investigators were focused on either the characteristics of nurses vis-à-vis death or on interventions to influence their anxiety, attitudes, or coping styles. The problems chosen for study in the 34 dissertations by nurses fell into four broad categories: nurses' attitudes and reactions to death, dying patients' responses and adaptations, educational influences on nurses' attitudes and behaviors, and the adaptations of family members to death and bereavement. Publications based on the dissertations by nurses were found for 14 of the 34.

METHODOLOGY AND THE STRUCTURE OF KNOWLEDGE

Observations on Methodology

Published studies on death-related matters of concern to nursing range from evaluation of demonstrations on home care without theoretical underpinnings (Kassakian, Bailey, Rinker, Stewart, & Yates, 1979; Martinson,

Armstrong, Geis, Anglim, Gronseth, MacInnis, Nesbit, & Kersey, 1978) to sophisticated efforts to use path analysis to create a causal model for explaining nurses' attitudes toward death and dying (Gow & Williams, 1977). Overall, the reviewed studies in death, dying, and terminal illness were not guided by a central paradigm. Rather they were fragmented pieces of research, somewhat variable in the quality of methods used and the stated relationships to established knowledge and theory. Some studies of nurses' reactions and attitudes toward death suffered from minimal attention to systematic methods (Bonine, 1967; Strank, 1972), validity and reliability (Martin & Collier, 1975), and investigator bias and response set (Hopping, 1977). Research on the influence of educational interventions on nurses' attitudes and behaviors ranged from those with an implied conceptual framework and no control for built-in bias (Snyder, Gertler, & Ferneau, 1973) to well conceptualized investigations showing careful attention to issues of design, sampling, and interpretation of results (Padilla, Baker, & Dolan, 1975). Other studies suffered from the lack of a control group (Laube, 1977) or inadequate operationalization of the treatments being tested (Hardesty, Note 2).

The theoretical frameworks and scientific methods in the studies reviewed were quite variable and reflected ties with other disciplines. Either explicitly or implicitly, the studies of nurses' attitudes and anxieties about death were predominantly psychological in orientation. Some made use of instruments developed by psychologists (Denton & Wisenbaker, 1977; Golub & Reznikoff, 1971); some were done in collaboration with psychologists (Hoggatt & Spilka, 1978–79; Lester, Getty, & Kneisl, 1974); some used methods with a psychological frame of reference (Yeaworth, Knapp, & Winget, 1974). An extension of this trend in attitude studies was the application of linguistic quantitative analysis to a search in taped interviews for indicators of avoidance (Mood & Lakin, 1979) and of denial (Mood & Lick, 1979).

Studies of patient, family, and nurse adaptations to death and dying were set in a variety of conceptual frameworks. These data were produced by many methods: participant observation (Quint, 1963), unstructured and semistructured interviews (Castles & Keith, 1979; Dubrey & Terrill, 1975; Hampe, 1975; Nash, 1979; Qvarnstrom, 1979), interviews using scales and scored instruments (Fitzpatrick, Donovan, & Johnston, 1980; Laborde & Powers, 1980; Lewis, 1982), Q-sort techniques (Freihofer & Felton, 1976; Irwin & Meier, 1973), questionnaires (Huckabay & Jagla, 1979; Niko-laisen & Williams, 1980), and a combination of methods (Lyall, Vachon, & Rogers, 1980; McCorkle, 1977). Examination of patterns of nurse-patient contacts and provider communication with patients was done using direct observation (Keck & Walther, 1977; Wegmann, 1979), questionnaires (Pienschke, 1973), reports of incidents by nurses (Hurley, 1977), and examination of medical records (McCorkle, 1978). Patients' records also served as data sources for descriptive analyses of reported patterns of dying in hospitals (Benoliel, 1977a, 1977b; Swenson, Matsura, & Martinson, 1979).

Early studies using statistical procedures were for the most part comparisons of central tendencies or rankings, and the reports varied in attention to detail and procedural controls. Some recent publications described the application of multiple regression techniques to investigations of nurses' responses to death (Stoller, 1980), cancer patient responses to psychosocial variables (McCorkle & Benoliel, Note 3), and adaptation to conjugal bereavement (Vachon, Rogers, Lyall, Lancee, Sheldon, & Freeman, 1982). In general, there has been an increase in methodological sophistication in the use of statistics since 1970. Content analysis was applied in the majority of studies using data obtained through interviews and participant observation. Descriptions of actual procedures in these studies ranged from reports in which content analysis was implied but not described (Price & Bergen, 1977; Simmons & Given, 1972) to those in which procedures for establishing categories, validity, and reliability were spelled out in detail (Castles & Murray, 1979; Martocchio, 1982; Degner, Beaton, & Glass, Note 4). Others described the process of data production but gave limited information about the creation of categories and their application to the data (Germain, 1979; Quint, 1966; Saunders, 1981; Spitzer & Folta, 1964). In general, precision in the reporting of qualitative analyses improved over the years. Research for the creation of theory on death and dying was influenced strongly by sociological thinking, particularly by the grounded theory methodology (Atwood, 1977; Degner & Glass, Note 5).

Observations on Mode of Inquiry and Knowledge Expansion

The information that has accumulated to date through nursing research in death, dying, and terminal illness is difficult to evaluate systematically because of the diversity in conceptual origins and the absence of an overriding paradigm. The bulk of published research has been descriptive in nature, some initiated by clinical observations and some posed within the context of established theoretical perspectives. Tying the pieces together into a coherent schema for nursing is difficult when some reported outcomes were nontheoretical, action-focused "facts" (Kassakian et al., 1979; Martinson, Armstrong, Geis, Anglim, Gronseth, MacInnis, Kersey, & Nesbit, 1978; Moldow & Martinson, 1980); some came out of derived conceptual frameworks (Laborde & Powers, 1980; Lewis, 1982); and others were based in established theories of crises (Demi, 1978; Williams & Nikolaisen, 1982), psychodynamic processes (Qvarnstrom 1979; Sanders, 1979), psychosocial transitions (Vachon, Formo, Freedman, Lyall, Rogers, & Freeman, 1976; McCorkle & Benoliel, Note 3), and symbolic interactionism (Quint, 1967). The paradigm-directed studies for the most part have been guided by theories and concepts developed in other disciplines. Some have contributed to the accumulation of knowledge about nurses' attitudes and responses to death (Fochtman, 1974; Martin, 1982–83; Ross, 1978; Stoller, 1980–81), the effects of death and dying on social roles and interactions (Hurley, 1977; Martocchio, 1982) and role expectations (Keith & Castles, 1979), factors affecting grief and bereavement (Benoliel, 1974; Sanders, 1979, 1979–80, 1980–81), and death influences on children's concepts and anxieties (Swain, 1979; Waechter, 1969, 1971).

Few explanatory and predictive studies were found. Quasi-experiments and other studies of nursing interventions fell into three areas: the education of nurses relative to death, dying, and bereavement; interventions to assist survivors in their adaptations to bereavement; and utilization of research findings to bring about changes in nursing practice. These studies varied considerably in the quality of conceptualization and instrumentation. Some suffered from problems in design (Constantino, 1981; Crowder, Yamamoto, & Simonowitz, 1976; Laube, 1977), bringing into question the validity of the findings. In contrast, the investigations of an in-service education program for nurses by Padilla et al. (1975, 1977), a course on death and grief by Miles (1980), and a self-help intervention program for widows by Vachon, Lyall, Rogers, Freedman-Letofsky, and Freeman (1980) were carefully planned and implemented and provide much food for thought. The reports by Dracup and Breu (1977, 1978) on the utilization of research findings about grieving spouses to bring about changes in hospital nursing practices illustrated the complexity of introducing applied research into an established social system.

In terms of types of knowledge—factual, conceptual, theoretical, and metatheoretical/methodological—nursing research on death, dying, and terminal illness has produced primarily factual knowledge and, to a lesser extent, conceptual knowledge (Atwood, 1978; Benoliel, 1971; Johnson-Soderberg, 1981). The generation of theories and models is in its infancy, and these efforts have their origins in sociological concepts and modes of inquiry (Degner et al., Note 4; Vachon, Note 6). Vachon's work on a model of adaptation to widowhood derives from her collaborative activities in a multidisciplinary research group (Vachon et al., 1980). In the metatheoretical/methodological realm, efforts have been directed mainly to the development of research instruments.

The earliest contribution to instrumentation was made by Folta (1965), who developed three scales for measuring the meaning of death, a sacred-secular orientation toward death, and anxiety relative to death. The scales showed reasonably good psychometric properties and were used initially to study the death attitudes of hospital nurses. Subsequently, Folta's attitude scales were used by Degner (1974) in a study of physicians' beliefs about life-prolonging decisions and by Gow and Williams (1977) in a multivariate study of factors affecting nurses' attitudes toward death. In 1975, Padilla et al. developed a Meaning of Death scale, using semantic differential techniques with 15 bipolar adjectives, and the scale was used in a series of studies testing the effects of education on nurses' attitudes toward death (Padilla et al., 1975).

Clinical observations stimulated the development and testing of a Symptom Distress Scale by McCorkle and Young (1978) and a Social Dependency Scale (Benoliel, McCorkle, & Young, 1980) to investigate changes in the responses of advanced cancer patients over time. These instruments were revised, retested, and strengthened in a later methodological study formulated to develop a battery of instruments for use in longitudinal investigations of advanced cancer patients' adaptations to living with the disease (McCorkle & Benoliel, Note 3). Both scales were found to have reasonable sensitivity, good psychometric properties, and potential for application to studies of other life-threatening illnesses.

In 1979, Sanders, Mauger, and Strong (Note 7) developed the Grief Experience Inventory (GEI) with 135 items covering seven content areas: somatic concerns, emotions, interpersonal relationships, thought content, funeral, religion, and denial. Psychometric properties have been reported and norms established for a general reference group and a newly bereaved group. The validity of the GEI has been tested using the Minnesota Multiphasic Personality Inventory (MMPI), and four groups—disturbed, depressed, denial, and normal—were identified showing distinct patterns in their scores on both instruments (Sanders, 1979). The GEI appears to have good potential for use in nursing research with various populations of bereaved individuals.

A quality of life instrument using linear analogue scales was designed for measurement of symptoms, capacity for daily activities, and estimates of life satisfaction in studies of cancer patients undergoing therapeutic clinical trials. It was tested initially on 15 patients, and test-retest of the scales within 24 hours on seven of the subjects showed a reproducibility of $r = .976$ by linear regression analysis (Presant, Klahr, & Hogan, 1981). The tool was subsequently revised to include 14 items covering side effects, daily activities, and general life satisfaction indicators and was tested on large samples of cancer patients, diabetic noncancer patients, and healthy individuals (Padilla, Presant, Grant, Baer, & Metter, 1981). Statistical testing of these data supported the instrument's potential for reproducibility in a high proportion of cases, as well as for construct validity of the three identified areas. Comparisons of patients' scores with physicians' estimates of quality of life produced poor correlations, suggesting that the instrument may be useful as a valid and reliable measure of quality of life from the patient's perspective.

SUBSTANTIVE CONTRIBUTIONS BY MAJOR AREA

The substantive contributions to nursing knowledge about death, dying, and terminal illness fall into three categories. These areas of concern center on (a) reactions and responses of nurses to death and terminal illness, (b) adaptations of patients and families to death and dying, and (c) environments and social processes affecting adaptations to death, terminal illness, and bereavement.

Nurses' Responses to Death and Terminal Illness

Attitudes toward Death and Terminal Care. Early descriptive studies of nurses' attitudes toward death sought to identify their salient characteristics in relation to environmental influences. In a comparative study of the attitudes of nursing personnel in three hospitals, Folta (1965) found the majority of respondents viewing death as peaceful, predictable, and natural, yet viewing it simultaneously with a high degree of anxiety. No significant differences were found by hospital, but staff nurses showed the highest levels of anxiety compared to nurses in other positions. Gow and Williams (1977) investigated the relative influence of work environment and personal characteristics on the death attitudes of nurses in community agencies as well as hospitals and reported similar findings. Anxiety was the strongest predictor of attitudes toward death, and type of work setting showed little independent effect. Age rather than position was viewed as the critical variable; the findings showed younger nurses with higher anxiety levels, poorer perceptions of caring for the dying, and more negative attitudes than older nurses.

That direct exposure to death may be an important influence on nurses' attitudes was supported by findings of Fochtman (1974) that pediatric nurses on terminal and nonterminal wards had different attitudes about prolongation of life and conversations with dying children. In an earlier study, Bonine (1967) reported that student nurses exposed to children's deaths described themselves as frightened, helpless, angry, and ambivalent. When nursing personnel in London were interviewed concerning their perceptions of care, the situations described by them as highly distressing were personal identification with the patient, unpleasant types of dying, changes in patients' physical appearance, and lack of clear policies on care. In a survey of nurses, Hoggatt and Spilka (1978–79) found half of the respondents feeling adequate and comfortable most of the time and 90 percent against the use of extreme measures in prolonging life. Denton and Wisenbaker (1977) sought to determine the effect of exposure to death on the death anxiety of nurses and found an inverse relationship. In their view, the confounding influences of age and work experience could not be overlooked, and exposure to death had to be considered a multidimensional variable.

The influence of nurses' attitudes on their beliefs and caregiving practices provided additional support for the variable nature of death work in nursing. Stoller (1980–81) studied nurses' responses to selected work situations and found fear of death showing little relationship to direct encounters with death. Fear of others' dying, on the other hand, was statistically significant in predicting responses to unstructured interactions with dying patients, although only a small portion of the variance was explained. The expectation that increased work experience would lead to coping strategies for handling uneasiness in difficult work situations was not supported for nurses in regard to interactions with dying patients (Stoller, 1980). These results are congruent with other findings that avoidance and denial are strategies used by nurses for coping with stressful work situations involving death (Martin, 1982–83; Mood & Lakin, 1979; Mood & Lick, 1979). Social desirability may also be a factor affecting nurses' attitudes toward some caregiving activities. In a study of nurses' attitudes toward home care in Minnesota, Martinson, Palta, and Rude (1977, 1978) found 90 % indicating willingness to care for dying adults at home and 80 % to care for children.

Education is thought to be a powerful influence on the development of death attitudes in student nurses, but the importance of prior socialization into the death values of society cannot be overlooked. A survey of nursing students and graduate nurses by Golub and Reznikoff (1971) on attitudes toward terminal illness, autopsy, suicide prevention, life maintenance efforts, and heart transplants showed remarkable similarities in the two groups; the major differences were on attitudes toward autopsy and life maintenance activities. The graduate nurses were more favorable than students to the use of autopsies, suggesting the influence of nursing education and exposure to the norms of scientific medicine. The students were more approving than the nurses of extensive life support efforts, implying perhaps that students' views of hospital care were influenced strongly by societal values favoring heroic medical activity.

In a comparative study of students and faculty, Lester et al. (1974) hypothesized that fears of death and dying would decrease with increased academic preparation. The results were in the predicted direction with two exceptions. First-year graduate students scored higher than senior undergraduates on fears of death/dying of self, and junior undergraduates had top scores on fear of death of others. Clinical experience was thought to be the major contributor to these differences. A survey by Hopping (1977) to test the effects of death-oriented courses on student nurses' attitudes showed no changes associated with the experience. In another study by Martin and Collier (1975), students self-reports indicated increased comfort, security, and willingness to talk about death at the time of final testing. When first-year and senior students in three- and four-year educational programs were studied for differences in attitudes associated with curriculum experiences, the findings showed a decrease in death ideation in the three-year school (Snyder et al., 1973) and an increase in flexibility and openness to communication with dying patients in the other (Yeaworth et al., 1974).

Although education is a likely contributor to the development of death attitudes and behaviors in nurses, the exact nature of that contribution is far from clear. Jinadu and Adediran (1982) compared the effects of nursing education on the death attitudes of first- and third-year students in Nigeria and found no significant differences between the groups. These findings are in contrast with those reported in similar studies in western societies and show the need for systematic investigations that take account of variations in direct exposure to death, cultural modes of managing dying, and educational practices.

The direct effect of education on outcomes for nurses has not been easy to determine. When fantasy and relaxation techniques were tested by Ross (1978) for their influence on nurses' responses to statements by dying patients, the results showed that the statistical differences between groups with high and low death concerns and sensitized and repressed death concerns were confounded by differences in age. Clarification of the complex relationships implied by these educational studies requires more rigorous research than has been demonstrated thus far.

Stress Responses of Nurses.   Death as a stressor for nurses has been identified in relation to critical care nursing, work with cancer patients, and investigators' experiences during research on death and dying. At least 19 studies of stresses experienced by nurses in critical care work have been done (Stehle, 1981). Death on a coronary care unit was reported as a stressful ambiguity as expressed in frustration over the organization of work and a sense of simultaneously doing too much and too little (Price & Bergen, 1977). When intensive care nurses from six different hospitals were surveyed by Huckabay and Jagla (1979) in relation to stressors in their work, the respondents ranked work load pressures, death of a patient, and communication problems among staff as first, second, and third in importance. Critical care work per se may not be the sole factor, however. In a military hospital (Maloney, 1982) found nonintensive care nurses reported more state anxiety, more somatic complaints, and greater dissatisfaction with workload than those on intensive care settings. In a review of critical care studies, Stehle (1981) summarized the state of the art in this area of research by noting that the majority of the studies substantiated the stressful nature of the work but suffered from a lack of attention to theoretical foundations, clear differentiation of structural and personal stresses, implementation of intervention strategies, and evaluation of interventions.

Studies of stress experienced in nursing work with advanced cancer patients revealed that the nurses focused on the problems of dying patients as a displacement for their own concerns (Vachon, Lyall, & Freeman, 1978). The experience of initiating a new palliative care unit was found by Vachon et al. (1978) to result in stress scores for the nurses that were twice those of nurses on other hospital units and close to those of new widows. Three months later, stress levels were still high for 50 % of the nurses, and factors contributing to the stresses were observed by the investigators to be both structural and personal (Lyall, et al., 1980). Six months later, the stress scores had decreased to normal levels on the average, but patterns of scapegoating and stereotyping among the staff were observed instead of open discussion about work difficulties (Lyall et al., 1980). These studies give evidence that the stresses in cancer work may well derive from a combination of circumstances including unrealistic expectations by the staff, structural conditions incompatible with the goals of the work, and personal characteristics of the staff. Further research is needed to clarify the nature of these complex relationships and to propose interventions to counteract those stresses that are amenable to change or attenuation.

The nature of support for nurses in stressful work arenas is an area in need of systematic investigation. The evidence available at this time shows mainly that physicians and nurses seek support in different ways. A survey of the professional staff giving home care to dying children provided evidence that the nurses relied on families, coworkers, support group sessions, and contacts with the project staff for support; in contrast, the physicians derived support mainly from reliance on self and physical activity (Gronseth, Martinson, Kersey, & Nesbit, 1981). Vachon et al. (1978) found that physicians responded to the availability of consultation for difficult patient situations, whereas nurses and social workers made use of support groups and meetings for discussion. The Baider and Porath (1981) study of the regular use of group sessions with nurses on a cancer ward in Israel gave evidence that this activity was useful in facilitating communication, consultation, and support among the nursing staff. Many of the stresses reported by nurses related to the structural conditions under which they worked, and the extent to which these can be altered is far from clear.

Investigation into problems of death and dying can also produce stresses for the nurse-investigator. These stresses have been associated with the strains of continuing contacts with dying patients (Quint, 1964); social isolation from peers and conflicts between nurse and investigator roles when the person collecting data occupies both positions (Benoliel, 1975); a sense of exploiting professional colleagues in the interest of collecting data (Martocchio, 1982); and ethical problems relative to decisions to intervene and on matters of confidentiality and privacy (Benoliel, 1975).

Patients' and Families' Adaptations to Death and Dying

The Meaning of Dying to Patients.   Patients' perspectives on death, dying, and terminal illness have been identified in investigations about cancer, quality of life, and the experience of hospitalization. An early longitudinal study on women's adaptations following mastectomy produced evidence that the women viewed their futures as uncertain (Quint, 1963), experienced a sense of isolation from others (Quint, 1964), and encountered many obstacles in their efforts to obtain information about extent of disease and prognosis (Quint, 1965). Family relationships and information control by physicians were identified by McCorkle (1977, 1978) as key factors affecting the adaptive patterns of individuals with nonresectable lung cancer during the period of terminal illness. In a comparative study of terminally ill cancer patients and controls on time dimensions, Fitzpatrick, Donovan, and Johnston (1980) found the cancer patients had shorter time projections and experienced more time pressures than control subjects even though they reported more free time. When Lewis (1982) tested the relationships of perceived control over life and over health to self-esteem, purpose in life, and anxiety in advanced cancer patients, perceived control over life showed statistically significant relationships with the three variables, as had been predicted. Unexpectedly, perceived control over health was associated significantly only with purpose in life, suggesting that health takes on a different meaning in terminal illness.

Further evidence that illness associated with the threat of death fosters changes in perceptions of self and life was provided by comparative studies of the effects of different chronic diseases. Subjects with severe osteoarthritis and end-stage renal disease were compared by Laborde and Powers (1980), using life satisfaction as a measure of quality of life. The groups were essentially the same on past and future relationships, but the patients on dialysis considered present life as better than the past, whereas the opposite view was held by those with arthritis. McCorkle and Benoliel (McCorkle, Benoliel, Mumma, Germino, Georgiadou, & Driever, 1982; McCorkle & Benoliel, Note 3) tested newly diagnosed patients with cancer or heart disease at one and two months following diagnosis with a battery of instruments, including measures of symptom distress, pain, and mood disturbance, to determine whether responses varied by disease and occasion. Mean differences showed cancer patients suffering more physical distress and mood disturbance on the average than patients with myocardial infarction at both occasions. The most striking finding was that both groups reported fewer concerns and better mood at the second interview even though physical distress remained much the same, suggesting that a process of threat assimilation had taken place. These studies suggest that continued investigation of the adaptive patterns associated with different forms of terminal disease is critical to the expansion of scientific knowledge about the impact of possible death on the daily lives of patients.

Hospitalized patients served as data sources for other studies about the meaning of dying. Simmons and Given (1972) found that the majority of terminal patients welcomed the opportunity to talk about their concerns if given the opportunity. In a study to determine whether dying patients experienced loneliness, Dubrey and Terrill (1975) found 35 out of 50 denying its existence. These respondents did not view the nurse as a source for emotional support and expected such assistance from family relationships. Similar findings were reported by Castles and Keith (1979), who found that hospitalized dying patients in a rural community defined their roles as conformity to established norms and expected their support from family and religion. Using a psychodynamic framework, Qvanstrom (1979) found patients oscillating between understanding and denial, depending on the situation, between acceptance and protest, and between hope and resignation. Nash (1979) used content analysis of interviews with 24 terminal patients to identify incidents in which treatment with dignity or without could be inferred and found 90% of the 126 incidents not congruent with respect for human dignity. These studies suggested that hospitalized dying patient's responses resulted from a complex interaction among personal, structural, and cultural variables. Sophisticated research is essential to unravel the complexity of these relationships.

Family Perspectives on Dying. Although less attention has been given to the perspectives of family members on dying, the investigations have been remarkable in the consistency of their findings. Irwin and Meier (1973) found that relatives in the hospital defined support by staff in two ways. They wanted (a) honest information and clear explanations relative to the dying person's condition and what was being done and (b) assurance that the staff was keeping the patient as comfortable as possible. Similar results were reported by Hampe (1975), in a study of grieving spouses, and by Freihofer and Felton (1976), whose sample consisted of relatives in a military hospital. The three analyses also identified nurses' behaviors the relatives reported as least supportive for them: efforts to (a) encourage them to cry, (b) remove them from the bedside of the patient, and (c) remind them that the suffering would be over soon. These findings implied discrepancies between nurses' and families' definitions of support and the need for systematic investigation of interventions helpful to families of hospitalized dying patients.

The adaptation of families to other facets of terminal illness is an area of serious neglect. Only one such study was found. Data from an interview performed one month after a husband's death were used by Vachon, Freedman, Formo, Rogers, Lyall, and Freeman (1977) to construct the widows' view of the final illness and to identify the influence of disease and husband-wife communication on these views. One set of women saw the final illness as terminal and leading to death, whereas the others defined it as "lingering" and were shocked when death occurred. Women who recalled communication with their husbands as movement back and forth between acceptance and denial appeared to have the most difficult transition, compared to those using open communication or mutual pretense. Type of disease was an important influence. The widows of cancer victims perceived the dying period as more stressful than did those whose husbands died of heart disease, and the former had many complaints about the medical care system. Prospective studies of family adaptations to terminal illness would appear to be a necessary step in the advancement of knowledge about the nature of family involvement in dying.

Childhood Views on Death.   A pioneer contribution to death research in nursing was made by Waechter (1969, 1971), who compared children having fatal illnesses with control groups of children. She found those with terminal disease having twice as much anxiety as the others and showing much concern with loneliness, separation, and death. The majority of the terminal group projected various forms of death imagery in their drawings and comments, suggesting thereby that they were picking up cues about their situation even though most parents did not talk openly to them. Swain (1979) interviewed children 2 through 16 years of age for their ideas about the finality of death, the inevitability of death, and open acknowledgment of death as a personal event. Only age was significant, and the greatest change in thinking took place between ages 5 and 7—suggesting the influence of other children through entry into school. Both studies pointed to the influence of social interaction on children's perceptions of death and dying. Continued nursing research on children's experiences with death and dying can broaden what is presently known about children's modes of coping with these major turning points in life.

Grief, Bereavement, and Widowhood.   Bereavement responses following the death of a spouse have been examined for variations in the age of the survivor at the time of death (Sanders, 1980–81; Vachon et al., 1976); premorbid personality characteristics (Sanders, 1979); adjustment following suicide (Demi, 1978); and type of death (Saunders, 1981). The evidence showed younger widows with higher grief intensities two months after death than older widows but with better adjustment on the average at 18 months when compared to the older group (Sanders, 1980–81). That age is important in early bereavement was further supported by Vachon et al. (1976), who found higher stress scores in women under 45 years of age than in those who were older. When widows were compared for adjustment after a husband's sudden death, Demi (1978) found no differences on measures of physical and mental health but a trend toward less satisfactory social adjustment for postsuicidal widows. According to Saunders' (1981) analysis, adjustment to widowhood by young women required a transformation in identity, and experiences with other people made crucial contributions to the direction of change. Adaptation to bereavement after the loss of a spouse cannot be viewed simplistically as age-related, according to the findings of Vachon et al. (1982). Their analysis showed that the best predictor of stress levels two years after the death was the score on the Goldberg General Health Questionnaire (Goldberg, Rickels, Downing, & Hesbacker, 1976) at one month after the death in combination with poor health before bereavement. The evidence to date suggests that healthy and unhealthy adaptations to widowhood come about through an interplay of personal and social variables, and sophisticated research to understand these complex relationships is essential for the discipline of nursing.

Loss of a child was found by Sanders (1979–80) to produce higher grief intensities in the survivors than either the loss of a spouse or parent. That mothers and fathers behave differently in response to the sudden loss of an infant was supported in a survey of parents whose child died of sudden infant death syndrome (Nikolaisen & Williams, 1980; Williams & Nikolaisen, 1982). The findings also showed that adaptation to the crisis of sudden infant loss was influenced by the parent's education, income, and marital status. Much remains to be learned about how families adapt to the loss of a child as a basis for planning nursing interventions. Increased attention to this area of research is highly recommended.

Environments, Social Processes, and Adaptations to Death

Congruence of Nurse-Patient Perceptions and Behaviors.   Evidence from hospitalized terminal patients and nurses showed different expectations for the groups about appropriate behavior for dying patients and nurses (Castles & Keith, 1979). The patients believed that dying patients should be and were cooperative. The nurses expected idiosyncratic behaviors from some dying patients, and they labeled a high percentage of actual behaviors by patients in this manner. Ironically, consensus on expectations for peers was greater among dying patients than among nurses, and the investigators hypothesized that the variations among nurses might derive from lack of clarity about the skills involved in care of the dying (Keith & Castles, 1979). When advanced cancer patients and their caregivers were compared by Jennings and Muhlenkamp (1981) for perceptions of patients' levels of anxiety, hostility, and depression, the results showed the caregivers' ratings of patients as worse on each affective state than the patients' themselves. In a comparison of health ratings by elderly bereaved persons and nurse interviewers, Valanis and Yeaworth (1982) found the subjects over 70 years old rating their physical health significantly better than did the nurses. The findings from these studies give evidence that nurses and patients use stereotypes in their appraisals of each other. Research to clarify how these tendencies influence the delivery of patient care could be highly informative.

Nurse-Patient Contacts and Communication. Evidence that a terminal diagnosis influenced the nature of nurse-patient interactions was reported by several investigators. Observations in a hospital by Keck and Walther (1977) produced findings that nurses spent more time with dying patients than with those not defined as dying, although no differences in emotional support could be identified. Similar results on the duration of nurse-patient contacts with terminal and nonterminal patients were reported by Wegmann (1979). She found, in addition, that despite more actual time with dying patients, the nurses used more verbal and nonverbal avoidance in their interactions with them than with patients who were not dying. In an analysis of nurse-patient incidents reported by nurses, Hurley (1977) also found that avoidance was the preferred coping strategy for nurses in their communications with dying patients. Pienschke (1973) gathered some evidence that physician openness about diagnosis and prognosis increased the nurses' effectiveness in giving care to hospitalized cancer patients, but the limitations in study design make these findings inconclusive. These results overall are congruent with the findings of Glaser and Strauss (1965) that avoidance by nurses functions as a protective strategy for maintaining composure under distressing work conditions.

Social Characteristics of Hospital Deaths. Descriptions of death as a hospital event were produced by investigators, using participant observation or content analysis of patient records. Spitzer and Folta (1964) found that expected deaths in the hospital were followed by a standardized pattern of communication unless a key person in the chain of information could not be located. Unexpected death produced nonstandardized patterns, increases in social interactions, and often disruptions in information flow. A retrospective analysis of hospital records by Benoliel (1977a) showed variations in treatment practices and patient characteristics by hospital; increases in active medical treatments and intensive care deaths between 1966 and 1971 (Benoliel, 1977b); and evidence that the amount of effort exerted to prolong life varied with underlying cause of dying, length of stay, and age (Mumma, 1981). In another record study, Swenson et al. (1979) observed that use of life sustaining treatments and cardiopulmonary resuscitation was overwhelmingly greater for patients with heart disease than for those with cancer. These findings reflect societal values promoting the use of biomedical technology. How nurses' behaviors relate to these variations in patterns of dying would seem an area worthy of systematic investigation.

Social Structure, Social Interaction, and Socialization.   The influence of social structure and social interaction was investigated in relation to the adaptations of patients, nurses, and student nurses. Quint (1965) produced evidence that institutionalized practices of information control by physicians and nurses served as obstacles for women after mastectomy to obtaining valid facts about their present and future situation. In another study, Quint (1966) reported that nurses on hospital wards with high death ratios encountered different kinds of death-related work problems and used different types of composure strategies, depending on the unit's primary work orientation and structural features. In another analysis, Quint (1967) described the socialization of student nurses to the meaning of work with dying patients as directly related to the ideology of the school, teachers' perspectives on death and dying, and the students' direct encounters with death and with dying patients. Students who learned to be relatively comfortable with dying patients had atypical experiences as students, including a mentor who provided guidance in death-related matters.

In an ethnographic description of a cancer ward, Germain (1979) showed the working atmosphere of the ward to be affected by physicians' conflicts and differences in treatment orientation, the personal crises of the nursing staff, and the anger of patients and families toward each other and care providers. One result was considerable role strain for the nurses. Martocchio (1982) used participant observation to identify patterns and processes that typify the social situation of the dying patient in the hospital. She analyzed the situation to be characterized by uncertainty and conflict resulting from (a) a recognition by staff of too many norms judged to be equal in value and (b) a continual search for structure, the use of bargains to establish rules of behavior, and ongoing negotiations among all participants to clarify roles and identities. The common denominator in these studies was a recognition that human responses to death and dying were influenced and altered by the context of interactions and by transactions with other people.

From three studies, theories were produced proposing relationships among social, structural, and process variables in terms of their influence on decisions and consequences for patients, families, and providers. Empirical data were used by Degner et al. (Note 4) to generate a theory of life-death decision making in health care. Relationships among the categories of organizational structure, availability of medical technology, types of control, and available knowledge were described in terms of hypothesized influences on decision making processes, interpersonal dynamics, and outcomes for life-threatened patients. In a study by Atwood (1977, 1978), selective neglect was identified as the central category for a theory of family views on perimortal nursing care. In the analysis, neglect was shown to explain discrepancies between role expectations and role performances by family members and staff in the hospital. A longitudinal study of widows provided the basis for a model of adaptation to bereavement, showing how social support might function to influence the process and outcomes of bereavement for women over a two-year period (Vachon, Note 6). These theoretical formulations point to the social nature of human responses to death-related situations and the importance of time and change in scientific investigations of terminal illness and bereavement.

SUMMARY, RESEARCH DIRECTIONS

Notwithstanding its fragmented nature, nursing research into death, dying, and terminal illness produced evidence that (a) planned social support can accelerate the adaptation of widows during bereavement (Vachon et al., 1980); (b) focused educational programs can contribute to changes in nurses' attitudes and knowledge about death and grief (Miles, 1980; Padilla et al., 1975, 1977); and (c) innovations in nursing practices can be facilitated when planned interventions take account of the social system of the work environment (Dracup & Breu, 1977, 1978). Findings from feasibility studies of nurses' contributions to home care programs for dying patients should be accepted with caution because control groups were not used and little attention was directed toward identifying the characteristics of families for whom the experience of dying at home might be most suitable (Kassakian et al., 1979; Martinson, Armstrong, Geis, Anglim, Gronseth, MacInnis, Kersey, & Nesbit, 1978; Martinson, Armstrong, Geis, Anglim, Gronseth, MacInnis, Nesbit, & Kersey, 1978). The assumption that home care is best needs to be tested under controlled conditions with attention to quality of life variables as well as to cost and a clear specification of nursing interventions. Evidence that the attitudes and behaviors of student nurses toward death and dying change during their basic educational experiences was found in a number of studies. Whether these changes result from the influence of formal programs or informal socialization is unclear, because control comparisons were not made. Longitudinal study to verify the validity of the implied relationship of educational experience to behavioral outcomes is needed.

The stressful nature of death and dying for patients, families, and nurses has been identified repeatedly; yet relatively little is known about what can be done to facilitate positive and productive adaptations to these stresses for the recipients and the providers of nursing services. Much also remains to be learned about the characteristics of high risk individuals and groups, meaning those with high vulnerability to unhealthy adaptations and outcomes in encounters with death and dying. According to Vachon (1982), variables to be considered include age, quality of family relationship, extreme avoidance behaviors, time in the life cycle, and availability of social support. The influence of variations in cultural beliefs and practices on adaptations to terminal illness and bereavement has received minimal attention. Demonstration and evaluation of modifications in work environments to facilitate the delivery of personalized nursing services before, during, and after the time of death are clearly needed.

For the discipline of nursing, the studies on death and dying point to the social nature of nursing transactions and the need to clarify the goals and operations of nursing practice in terminal illness. Limited scientific knowledge is available about the nature of social support useful to people undergoing major transitions associated with death and dying and the variations in support required depending on personal characteristics, temporal points in the transition, and contextual variables (Walker, MacBride, & Vachon, 1977). The theories and models produced to date provide direction for the testing of hypotheses in future research. The concepts of group loss and multiple losses (Benoliel, 1971), selective neglect (Atwood, 1977, 1978), risk-benefit calculations in decision making (Degner & Glass, Note 5), and grief themes of families (Johnson-Soderberg, 1981) are potential sources of influence for other studies in the field. Despite these contributions, the outcomes overall show the need for paradigm-directed nursing research with a sound integration of central concepts and research methods, if systematic knowledge about the meanings of death, dying, and terminal illness is to move forward. The results also suggest that the improvement of nursing services for dying patients and their families requires that serious attention be given by leaders in nursing to changes in structural conditions affecting how nurses practice and to the use of available knowledge about the concerns and needs of dying patients and their families. It would appear that nurses' actions that encourage consumers to talk about their feelings need to be replaced with more helpful forms of nursing intervention.

REFERENCE NOTES

1. Kalish & Kastenbaum (Eds.). *Omega: A newsletter concerned with time perspective, death and bereavement,* 1966, *1.*
2. Hardesty, F. The relative effectiveness of three methods of teaching student nurses the psychology of grief and mourning. *Science and direct patient care: II.* Papers presented at the fifth annual Nurse Scientist Conference. Denver, Colo.: University of Colorado School of Nursing, April 1972.
3. McCorkle, R., & Benoliel, J. Q. *Cancer patient responses to psychosocial variables.* Unpublished report. Seattle: University of Washington, Community Health Care Systems Department, 1981. (Available at cost from Ruth McCorkle, Ph.D., Community Health Care Systems Department, University of Washington, Seattle, Washington 98195.)
4. Degner, L. F., Beaton, J. I., & Glass, H. P. *Life-death decision making in health care: A descriptive theory.* Unpublished report. Winnipeg, Manitoba: University of Manitoba School of Nursing, 1981.
5. Degner, L. F., & Glass, H. P. Calculations of risk versus benefit: Indicators of health care decision making. In G. N. Zilm, S. M. Stinson, M. E. Steed, & P. Overton (Eds.), *Development and use of indicators in nursing research, proceedings of the 1975 National Conference on Nursing Research.* Edmonton, Alberta: University of Alberta School of Nursing, 1975.
6. Vachon, M. L. S. *The importance of social relationships and social support in widowhood.* Unpublished report, 1980. (Available from Mary L. S. Vachon, Ph.D., Clarke Institute of Psychiatry, 250 College Street, Toronto, Ontario M5T 1R8, Canada.)
7. Sanders, C. M., Mauger, P. A., & Strong, P. N. *A manual for the grief experience inventory.* Unpublished report, 1979. (Available at cost from Catherine M. Sanders, Ph.D., Suite 423, Doctors Building, 1012 South Kings Drive, Charlotte, North Carolina 28283.)

REFERENCES

Anthony, S. *The child's discovery of death.* New York: Harcourt, 1940.
Atwood, J. R. A grounded theory approach to the study of perimortality care. In M. V. Batey (Ed.), *Communicating nursing research* (Vol. 9). Boulder, Colo: Western Interstate Commission for Higher Education, 1977.

Atwood, J. R. The phenomenon of selective neglect. In E. Bauwens (Ed.), *The anthropology of health.* St Louis: Mosby, 1978.

Baider, L., & Porath, S. Uncovering fear: Group experience of nurses in a cancer ward. *International Journal of Nursing Studies,* 1981, *18,* 47–52.

Bendann, E. *Death customs: An analytical study of burial rites.* New York: Alfred A. Knopf, 1930.

Benedict, R. *Patterns of culture.* Boston: Houghton-Mifflin, 1934.

Benoliel, J. Q. Assessments of loss and grief. *Journal of Thanatology,* 1971, *1,* 182–194.

Benoliel, J. Q. Anticipatory grief in physicians and nurses. In B. Schoenberg, A. C. Carr, A. H. Kutscher, D. Peretz, & I. K. Goldberg (Eds.), *Anticipatory grief.* New York: Columbia University Press, 1974.

Benoliel, J. Q. Research related to death and the dying patient. In P. J. Verhonick (Ed.), *Nursing research I.* Boston: Little, Brown, 1975.

Benoliel, J. Q. Social characteristics of death as a recorded hospital event. In M. V. Batey (Ed.), *Communicating nursing research* (Vol. 8). Boulder, Colo.: Western Interstate Commission for Higher Education, 1977. (a)

Benoliel, J. Q. A comparison of technological influences on dying characteristics in one hospital during 1966 and 1971. In M. V. Batey (Ed.), *Communicating nursing research* (Vol. 10). Boulder, Colo.: Western Interstate Commission for Higher Education, 1977. (b)

Benoliel, J. Q. The changing social context for life and death decisions. *Essence,* 1978, *2,* 5–14.

Benoliel, J. Q., McCorkle, R., & Young, K. Development of a social dependency scale. *Research in Nursing and Health,* 1980, *3,* 3–10.

Blauner, R. Death and social structure. *Psychiatry,* 1966, *29,* 378–394.

Blumberg, J. E., & Drummond, E. E. *Nursing care of the long-term patient.* New York: Springer, 1963.

Bonine, G. N. Students' reactions to children's deaths. *American Journal of Nursing,* 1967, *67,* 1439–1440.

Bowlby, J. Grief and mourning in infancy and early childhood. In *Psychoanalytic Study of the Child* (Vol. 15). New York: International Universities Press, 1960.

Bruce, S. J. Reactions of mothers and nurses to stillbirths. *Nursing Outlook,* 1962, *10,* 88–91.

Buckeridge, A. J., Geiser, M. L., & Thomas, B. J. A study of overt nurse action when Darvon and Darvon compound are prescribed for p.r.n. administration. *Convention clinical sessions* (Vol. 3). New York: American Nurses Association, 1964.

Castles, M. R., & Keith, P. M. Patient concerns, emotional resources, and perception of nurse and patient roles. *Omega,* 1979, *10,* 27–33.

Castles, M. R., & Murray, R. B. *Dying in an institution: Nurse/patient perspectives.* New York: Appleton-Century-Crofts, 1979.

Choron, J. *Death and western thought.* New York: Collier-Macmillan, 1963.

Constantino, R. E. Bereavement crisis intervention for widows in grief and mourning. *Nurse Research,* 1981, *30,* 351–353.

Crowder, J. E., Yamamoto, J., & Simonowitz, J. Training registered nurses as bereavement counselors in an occupational health service. *Hospital and Community Psychiatry,* 1976, 27, 851–852.

Degner, L. The relationship between some beliefs held by physicians and their life prolonging decisions. *Omega,* 1974, *5,* 223–232.

Demi, A. S. Adjustment to widowhood after a sudden death: Suicide and non-suicide survivors compared. In *Communicating nursing research* (Vol. 11). Boulder, Colo.: Western Interstate Commission for Higher Education, 1978.

Denton, J. A., & Wisenbaker, V. B. Death experience and death anxiety among nurses and nursing students. *Nursing Research,* 1977, *26,* 61–64.

Directory of nurses with doctoral degrees (ANA Publication No. G-143 6M 8/80). Kansas City, Mo.: American Nurses' Association, 1980.

Dracup, K. A., & Breu, C. S. Strengthening practice through research utilization. In M. V. Batey (Ed.), *Communicating nursing research* (Vol. 10). Boulder, Colo.: Western Interstate Commission for Higher Education, 1977.

Dracup, K., & Breu, C. S. Using nursing research findings to meet the needs of grieving spouses. *Nursing Research,* 1978, *27,* 212–216.

Dubrey, R. J., & Terrill, L. A. The loneliness of the dying person: An exploratory study. *Omega,* 1975, *6,* 357–371.

Eissler, K. R. *The psychiatrist and the dying patient.* New York: International Universities Press, 1955.

Eliot, T. D. The adjustive behavior of bereaved families: A new field for research. *Social Forces,* 1930, *8,* 543–549.

Eliot, T. D. A step toward the social psychology of bereavement. *Journal of Abnormal and Social Psychology,* 1933, *27,* 114–115.

Feifel, H. (Ed.). *The meaning of death.* New York: McGraw-Hill, 1959.

Fitzpatrick, J. J., Donovan, M. J., & Johnston, R. L. Experience of time during the crisis of cancer. *Cancer Nursing,* 1980, *3,* 191–194.

Fochtman, D. A comparative study of pediatric nurses' attitudes toward death. *Life-Threatening Behavior,* 1974, *4,* 107–117.

Folta, J. R. The perception of death. *Nursing Research,* 1965, *14,* 232–235.

Foundation of thanatology. *Journal of the American Medical Association,* 1968, *205,* 35.

Frazier, J. G. *The belief in immortality and the worship of the dead* (3 vols.). London: Macmillan & Company, 1913–1922.

Freihofer, P., & Felton, G. Nursing behaviors in bereavement: An exploratory study. *Nursing Research,* 1976, *25,* 332–336.

Freud, S. *Thoughts for the time on war and death* (Vol. 14). London: Hogarth Press, 1915.

Freud, S. *Beyond the pleasure principle* (Vol. 18). London: Hogarth Press, 1920.

Fulton, R. L. The clergyman and the funeral director: A study on role conflict. *Social Forces,* 1961, *39,* 317–323.

Fulton, R. (Ed.). *Death and identity.* New York: Wiley, 1965.

Germain, C. P. H. *The cancer unit: An ethnography.* Wakcfield, Mass.: Nursing Resources, Inc., 1979.

Glaser, B. G. & Strauss, A. L. *Awareness of dying.* Chicago: Aldine, 1965.

Glaser, B. G. & Strauss, A. L. *Time for dying.* Chicago: Aldine, 1968.

Goldberg, D. P., Rickels, K., Downing, R., & Hesbacker, P. A comparison of two psychiatric screening tests. *British Journal of Psychiatry,* 1976, *129,* 61–67.

Golub, S., & Reznikoff, M. Attitudes toward death: A comparison of nursing students and graduate nurses. *Nursing Research,* 1971, *20,* 503–508.

Gorer, G. The pornography of death. In W. Phillips & P. Rahv (Eds.), *Modern writing*. New York: Berkeley, 1956.

Gorer, G. *Death, grief and mourning*. New York: Doubleday, 1965.

Gow, C. M., & Williams, J. I. Nurses' attitudes toward death and dying: A causal interpretation. *Social Science and Medicine*, 1977, *11*, 191–198.

Gronseth, E. C., Martinson, I. M., Kersey, J. H., & Nesbit, M. E. Support system of health professionals as observed in the project of home care for the child with cancer. *Death Education*, 1981. *5*, 37–50.

Habenstein, R. W., & Lamers, W. M. *The history of American funeral directing*. Milwaukee: Bulfin, 1955.

Habenstein, R. W., & Lamers, W. M. *Funeral customs the world over*. Milwaukee: Bulfin, 1960.

Hampe, S. O. Needs of the grieving spouse in a hospital setting. *Nursing Research*, 1975, *24*, 113–120.

Hinton, J. M. *Dying*. Baltimore: Penguin Books, 1967.

Hoggatt, L., & Spilka, B. The nurse and the terminally ill patient: Some perspectives and projected actions. *Omega*, 1978–79, *9*, 255–266.

Hopping, B. L. Nursing students' attitudes toward death. *Nursing Research*, 1977, *26*, 443–447.

Huckabay, L. M. D., & Jagla, B. Nurses' stress factors in the intensive care unit. *Journal of Nursing Administration*, 1979, *9*(2), 21–26.

Hurley, B. A. Problems of interaction between nurses and dying patients: Certainty of death. In M. V. Batey (Ed.), *Communicating nursing research* (Vol. 9). Boulder, Colo.: Western Interstate Commission for Higher Education, 1977.

Irwin, B. L., & Meier, J. R. Supportive measures for relatives of the fatally ill. In M. V. Batey (Ed.), *Communicating nursing research* (Vol. 6). Boulder, Colo.: Western Interstate Commission for Higher Education, 1973.

Jennings, B. M., & Muhlenkamp, A. F. Systematic misperceptions: Oncology patients' self-reported affective states and their caregivers' perceptions. *Cancer Nursing*, 1981, *4*, 485–489.

Jinadu, M. K., & Adediran, S. O. Effects of nursing education on attitudes of nursing students toward dying patients in the Nigerian sociocultural environment. *International Journal of Nursing Studies*, 1982, *19*, 21–27.

Johnson-Soderberg, S. Grief themes. *Advances in Nursing Science*, 1981, *3*(4), 15–26.

Kalish, R. A. Some variables in death attitudes. *Journal of Social Psychology*, 1963, *59*, 137–145.

Kassakian, M. G., Bailey, L. H., Rinker, M., Stewart, C. A., & Yates, J. W. The cost and quality of dying: A comparison of home and hospital. *Nurse Practitioner*, 1979, *4*, 18–23.

Keck, V. E., & Walther, L. S. Nurse encounters with dying and nondying patients. *Nursing Research*, 1977, *26*, 465–469.

Keith, P. M., & Castles, M. R. Expected and observed behavior of nurses and terminal patients. *International Journal of Nursing Studies*, 1979, *16*, 21–28.

Koestenbaum, P. The vitality of death. *Journal of Existentialism*, 1964, *18*, 139–166.

Kroeber, A. L. Disposal of the dead. *American Anthropologist*, 1927, *29*, 308–315.

Kubler-Ross, E. *On death and dying*. New York: Macmillan, 1969.

Kyle, M. W. The nurse's approach to the patient attempting to adjust to inoperable cancer. In *Convention clinical sessions* (Vol. 8). New York: American Nurses' Association, 1964.

Laborde, J. M., & Powers, M. J. Satisfaction with life for patients undergoing hemodialysis and patients suffering from osteoarthritis. *Research in Nursing and Health*, 1980, *3*, 19–24.

Laube, J. Death and dying workshop for nurses: Its effect on their death anxiety level. *International Journal of Nursing Studies*, 1977, *14*, 111–120.

Lester, D., Getty, K., & Kneisl, C. R. Attitudes of nursing students and nursing faculty toward death. *Nursing Research*, 1974, *23*, 50–53.

Lewis, F. M. Experienced personal control and quality of life in late-stage cancer patients. *Nursing Research*, 1982, *31*, 113–119.

Lifton, R. J. *Death in life: Survivors of Hiroshima*. New York: Random House, 1968.

Lindemann, E. Symptomatology and management of acute grief. *American Journal of Psychiatry*, 1944, *101*, 141–148.

Lyall, A., Vachon, M., & Rogers, J. A study of the degree of stress experienced by professionals caring for dying patients. In I. Ajemian & B. M. Mount (Eds.), *R. V. H. Manual on palliative/hospice care*. New York: Arno Press, 1980.

Maloney, J. P. Job stress and its consequences on a group of intensive care and nonintensive care nurses. *Advances in Nursing Science*, 1982, *4*(2), 31–42.

Marris, P. *Widows and their families*. London: Routledge, 1958.

Martin, L. B., & Collier, P. A. Attitudes toward death: A survey of nursing students. *Journal of Nursing Education*, 1975, *14*(1), 28–35.

Martin, T. O. Death anxiety and social desirability among nurses. *Omega*, 1982–83, *13*, 51–58.

Martinson, I. M., Armstrong, G. D., Geis, D. P., Anglim, M. A., Gronseth, E. C., MacInnis, H., Kersey, J. H., & Nesbit, M. E. Home care for children dying of cancer. *Pediatrics*, 1978, *62*, 106–113.

Martinson, I. M., Armstrong, G. D., Geis, D. P., Anglim, M. A. Gronseth, E. C., MacInnis, H., Nesbit, M. E., & Kersey, J. H. Facilitating home care for children dying of cancer. *Cancer Nursing*, 1978, *1*, 41–45.

Martinson, I. M., Palta, M., & Rude, N. Death and dying: Selected attitudes and experiences of Minnesota's registered nurses. In M. V. Batey (Ed.), *Communicating nursing research* (Vol. 9). Boulder, Colo.: Western Interstate Commission for Higher Education, 1977.

Martinson, I. M., Palta, M., & Rude, N. V. Death and dying: Selected attitudes of Minnesota's registered nurses. *Nursing Research*, 1978, *27*, 226–229.

Martocchio, B. O. *Living while dying*. Bowie, Md.: Brady, 1982.

McCorkle, R. Terminal illness: Human attachments and intended goals. In M. V. Batey (Ed.), *Communicating nursing research* (Vol. 9). Boulder, Colo.: Western Interstate Commission for Higher Education, 1977.

McCorkle, R. Patient contacts with physicians during terminal illness. *Essence*, 1978, *2*, 25–34.

McCorkle, R., Benoliel, J. Q., Mumma, C. A., Germino, B., Georgiadou, F., & Driever, M. J. Cancer patient responses to psychosocial variables. In *Com-*

municating nursing research (Vol 15). Boulder, Colo.: Western Interstate Commission for Higher Education, 1982. (Abstract)

McCorkle, R., & Young, K. Development of a symptom distress scale. *Cancer Nursing*, 1978, *1*, 373–378.

Mieding, C. Differential characteristics of pain. In *Convention clinical sessions* (Vol. 10). New York: American Nurses' Association, 1964.

Miles, M. S. The effects of a course on death and grief on nurses' attitudes toward dying patients and death. *Death Education*, 1980, *4*, 245–260.

Moldow, D. G., & Martinson, I. M. From research to reality—home care for the dying child. *Maternal-Child Nursing*, 1980, *5*, 159–166.

Mood, D. W., & Lakin, B. A. Attitudes of nursing personnel toward death and dying: I. Linguistic indicators of avoidance. *Research in Nursing and Health*, 1979, *2*, 53–60.

Mood, D. W., & Lick, C. F. Attitudes of nursing personnel toward death and dying: II. Linguistic indicators of denial. *Research in Nursing and Health*, 1979, *2*, 95–99.

Mumma, C. M. Care, cure, and hospital dying trajectories. In *Communicating nursing research* (Vol. 14). Boulder, Colo.: Western Interstate Commission for Higher Education, 1981. (Abstract)

Nash, M. L. Dignity of person in the final phase of life—an exploratory study. *Omega*, 1979, *8*, 71–80.

Nikolaisen, S. M., & Williams, R. A. Patients' view of support following the loss of their infant to sudden infant death syndrome. *Western Journal of Nursing Research*, 1980, *2*, 593–601.

Norris, C. M. The nurse and the dying patient. *American Journal of Nursing*, 1955, *55*, 1214–1217.

Padilla, G. V., Baker, V. E., & Dolan, V. A. *Interacting with dying patients: An interhospital nursing research and nursing education project*. Duarte, Calif.: City of Hope National Medical Center, 1975.

Padilla, G. V., Baker, V. E., & Dolan, V. Interacting with dying patients. In M. V. Batey (Ed.), *Communicating nursing research* (Vol. 8). Boulder, Colo.: Western Interstate Commission for Higher Education, 1977.

Padilla, G., Presant, C. A., Grant, M., Baer, C., & Metter, G. Assessment of quality of life (QL) in cancer patients. *Proceedings of the American Association for Cancer Research*, 1981, *22*, 397. (Abstract)

Peplau, H. E. *Interpersonal relations in nursing*. New York: G. P. Putnam's Sons, 1952.

Pienschke, D. Guardedness or openness on the cancer unit. *Nursing Research*, 1973, *22*, 484–490.

Presant, C. A., Klahr, C., & Hogan, L. Evaluating quality of life in oncology patients: Pilot observations. *Oncology Nursing Forum*, 1981, *8*(3), 26–30.

Price, T. R., & Bergen, B. J. The relationship of death as a source of stress for nurses on a coronary care unit. *Omega*, 1977, *8*, 229–238.

Quint, J. C. The impact of mastectomy. *American Journal of Nursing*, 1963, *63*, 88–92.

Quint, J. C. The first year after mastectomy: The patients and the nurse researchers. In *Convention clinical session* (Vol. 9). New York: American Nurses' Association, 1964.

Quint, J. C. Institutionalized practices of information control. *Psychiatry*, 1965, *28*, 119–132.

Quint, J. C. Awareness of death and the nurse's composure. *Nursing Research*, 1966, *15*, 49–55.

Quint J. C. *The nurse and the dying patient*. New York: Macmillan, 1967.

Qvarnstrom, U. Patients' reactions to impending death. *International Nursing Review*, 1979, *26*, 117–119.

Ross, C. W. Nurses' personal death concerns and responses to dying patients' statements. *Nursing Research*, 1978, *27*, 64–68.

Sanders, C. M. The use of the MMPI in assessing bereavement outcome. In C. Newmark (Ed.), *MMPI: Clinical and research trends*. New York: Praeger, 1979.

Sanders, C. M. A comparison of adult bereavement on the death of a spouse, child and parent. *Omega*, 1979–80, *10*, 303–322.

Sanders, C. M. Comparison of younger and older spouses in bereavement outcomes. *Omega*, 1980–81, *11*, 217–232.

Santora, J. C. Bibliography of death and dying: A guide to doctoral dissertations of the 1970s, A-H. *Death Education*, 1980, *3*, 415–423. (a)

Santora, J. C. Bibliography of death and dying: A guide to doctoral dissertations of the 1970s, I-Z. *Death Education*, 1980, *4*, 100–109. (b)

Saunders, C. The moment of truth: Care of the dying person. In L. Pearson (Ed.), *Death and dying*. Cleveland: Case Western Reserve University Press, 1969.

Saunders, J. M. A process of bereavement resolution: Uncoupled identity. *Western Journal of Nursing Research*, 1981, *3*, 319–322.

Simmons, S., & Given, B. Nursing care of the terminal patient. *Omega*, 1972, *3*, 217–225.

Snyder, M., Gertler, R., & Ferneau, E. Changes in nursing students' attitudes toward death and dying: A measurement of curriculum integration effectiveness. *International Journal of Social Psychiatry*, 1973, *19*, 294–298.

Spitzer, S. P., & Folta, J. R. Death in the hospital: A problem for study. *Nursing Forum*, 1964, *3*(4), 85–92.

Stehle, J. L. Critical care nursing stress: The findings revisited. *Nursing Research*, 1981, *30*, 182–186.

Stoller, E. P. Effect of experience on nurses' responses to dying and death in a hospital setting. *Nursing Research*, 1980, *29*, 35–38.

Stoller, E. P. The impact of death-related fears on attitudes of nurses in a hospital work setting. *Omega*, 1980–81, *11*, 85–96.

Strank, R. A. Caring for the chronic sick and dying: A study of attitudes. *Nursing Times*, 1972, *68*, 166–169.

Sudnow, D. *Passing on: The social organization of dying*. Englewood Cliffs, N.J.: Prentice-Hall, 1967.

Swain, H. L. Childhood views of death. *Death Education*, 1979, *2*, 341–358.

Swenson, E., Matsura, J., & Martinson, I. M. Effects of resuscitation for patients with metastatic cancers and chronic heart disease. *Nursing Research*, 1979, *28*, 151–153.

Toynbee, R., Mant, A. K., Smart, N., Hinton, J., Yudkin, S., Rhode, E., Heywood, R., & Price, H. H. *Man's concern with death*. London: Hodder and Stoughton, 1968.

Ujhely, G. B. *The nurse and her problem patients.* New York: Springer, 1963.

Vachon, M. L. S. Grief and bereavement: The family's experience before and after death. In I. Gentles (Ed.), *Care for the dying and the bereaved.* Toronto: Toronto Anglican Book Centre, 1982.

Vachon, M. L. S., Formo, A., Freedman, K., Lyall, W. A. L., Rogers, J., & Freeman, S. J. J. Stress reactions in bereavement. *Essence,* 1976, *1*, 23–33.

Vachon, M. L. S., Freedman, K., Formo, A., Rogers, J., Lyall, W. A. L., & Freeman, S. J. J. The final illness in cancer: The widow's perspective. *Canadian Medical Association Journal,* 1977, *117*, 1151–1154.

Vachon, M. L. S., Lyall, W. A. L., & Freeman, S. J. J. Measurement and management of stress in health professionals working with advanced cancer patients. *Death Education,* 1978, *6*, 365–375.

Vachon, M. L. S., Lyall, W. A. L., Rogers, J., Freedman-Letofsky, K., & Freeman, S. J. J. A controlled study of self-help intervention for widows. *American Journal of Psychiatry,* 1980, *137*, 1380–1384.

Vachon, M. L. S., Rogers, J., Lyall, W. A., Lancee, W. J., Sheldon, A. R., & Freeman, S. J. J. Predictors and correlates of high distress in adaptation to conjugal bereavement. *American Journal of Psychiatry,* 1982, *139*, 998–1002.

Valanis, B. G., & Yeaworth, R. Ratings of physical and mental health in the older bereaved. *Research in Nursing and Health,* 1982, *5*, 137–146.

Volkart, E. M., & Michael, S. T. Bereavement and mental health. In A. H. Leighton, J. A. Clausen, & R. N. Wilson (Eds.), *Explorations in social psychiatry.* New York: Basic Books, 1957.

Waechter, E. H. Death anxiety in children with fatal illness. *Fifth nursing research conference.* New York: American Nurses' Association, 1969.

Waechter, E. H. Children's awareness of fatal illness. *American Journal of Nursing,* 1971, *71*, 1168–1172.

Walker, K. N., MacBride, A., & Vachon, M. L. S. Social support networks and the crisis of bereavement. *Social Science and Medicine,* 1977, *11*, 35–41.

Wegmann, J. A. Avoidance behaviors of nurses as related to cancer diagnosis and/or terminality. *Oncology Nursing Forum,* 1979, *6*(3), 8–14.

Weisman, A., & Hackett, T. Predilection to death: Death and dying as a psychiatric problem. *Psychosomatic Medicine,* 1961, *23*, 232–256.

Williams, R. A., & Nikolaisen, S. M. Sudden infant death syndrome: Parents' perceptions and responses to the loss of their infant. *Research in Nursing and Health,* 1982, *5*, 55–61.

Worcester, A. *Care of the aged, the dying and the dead.* Springfield, Ill: Charles C Thomas, 1935.

Yeaworth, R., Knapp, F. T., & Winget, C. Attitudes of nursing students toward the dying patient. *Nursing Research,* 1974, *23*, 20–24.

PART II

Research on Nursing Care Delivery

Nursing Staff Turnover, Stress, and Satisfaction: Models, Measures, and Management

ADA SUE HINSHAW

AND

JAN R. ATWOOD

COLLEGE OF NURSING AND UNIVERSITY HOSPITAL
ARIZONA HEALTH SCIENCES CENTER, TUCSON

CONTENTS

Staff turnover, stress, and satisfaction are continual problems plaguing the delivery of health care and, specifically, nursing care. Numerous investigations have been conducted to identify the major phenomena pertaining to these concerns. Models have been constructed and tested specifying the relationships among staff stress, satisfaction, other predictive factors, and voluntary/involuntary turnover. Traditionally, turnover has been the focus of research endeavors, while the other factors have been investigated in terms of their impact on it (Mobley, Griffeth, Hand, & Meglino, 1979).

Turnover of nursing staff, especially professional or registered nurses, merits attention because of its consequences in terms of quality of care compromises and economic costs. Just as the productivity and effectiveness of industrial organizations are decreased by personnel turnover, the delivery of quality nursing care in service organizations is compromised from the instability of continual nursing staff terminations (Consolvo, 1979; Wolf, 1981). Price (1977) cited several investigations of the effect of turnover on the delivery of nursing care, such as greater incidence of suicides in a mental health agency (Kahne, 1968) and a slower discharge of patients (Revans, 1964). A continual process of orienting nursing staff would lead to difficulties in organizing care, interpreting and individualizing care policies, and responding swiftly in emergencies. The monetary costs of staff turnover were cited by numerous authors (Consolvo, 1979; Donovan, 1980; Wolf, 1981). The orientation costs for a professional nurse entering an acute care agency averages about $2,000, not considering the six months of lower productivity that occurs with new employees.

The purpose of this chapter on intraorganizational factors is to summarize and critique the major investigations of nursing staff turnover. Job stress and satisfaction are discussed extensively as well, due to their dominance in the professional nursing literature and their relationships to turnover and nursing staff retention.

STAFF TURNOVER

Turnover can be defined as both an organizational and individual phenomenon. In this chapter, the focus will be on individual turnover. In the studies reviewed, individual turnover usually was defined as an individual terminating employment with an agency. Price (1977, p.4) defined turnover as the "the degree of individual movement across the membership boundary of a social system." Generally, in the research, the social system was considered an agency.

Two major types of turnover were considered: voluntary and involuntary. Voluntary turnover was defined as an individual initiating termination or quitting an agency; involuntary turnover was defined as the organization initiating the turnover or dismissing the employee (Price, 1977; Seybolt, Pavett, & Walker, 1978). Voluntary termination was the focus of most studies reviewed. Individual turnover, both voluntary and involuntary, was generally indexed through longitudinal investigations in which the number of months in an agency or the number of months from a designated survey were measured (Price & Mueller, 1981; Seybolt et al., 1978; Weisman, Alexander, & Chase, 1981).

Models for Turnover

Numerous multistage models were evident in the organizational, hospital management, and nursing literature and delineated factors that predicted turnover of professional and nonprofessional staff in health care or service organizations. In these models, research was synthesized concerning staff turnover, stress, and satisfaction. Several theoretical models illustrating the major types of theories concerning turnover are summarized here (Table 1). Only models that described nursing staff (registered nurses, licensed practical nurses, and/or nurses' aides) turnover are discussed.

The content of the models illustrated the complex, multivariate, multistaged nature of the problem of predicting actual nursing staff turnover. The models were causal in nature with clearly specified relationships among the factors, implying a well developed body of research knowledge from which to consider the issue of turnover. Several factors were similar across the models. For example, most of the models contained factors acknowledging the effect of mobility and job satisfaction on turnover.

The models differed on several major issues. Several models were more comprehensive than others, consisting of environmental, organizational, and individual characteristics (Price, 1977; Price & Mueller, 1981; Weisman, Alexander, & Chase, 1981); others were narrower in perspective, studying only individual characteristics (Hinshaw & Atwood, 1982; Seybolt et al., 1978). The more comprehensive models have a more organizational, structural approach to turnover, while the individual models were more social-psychological in nature.

The Professional Turnover (Price & Mueller, 1981), Professional Autonomy and Turnover (Weisman, Alexander, & Chase, 1981), and Anticipated Turnover (Hinshaw & Atwood, 1982) models contained factors aimed at identifying a potential for turnover: intent to stay, intent to leave, and anticipated turnover respectively. For Price and Mueller (1981) and Weisman, Alexander, and Chase (1981), the intent to stay and intent to leave factors indexed the level of individual commitment to the organization (Mobley et al. 1979). For Hinshaw and Atwood (1982), anticipated turnover allowed for the assessment and possible prevention of nursing

Table 1. Models for Turnover.

Model/author(s)	Characteristics of model	Initial stage factors	Intervening stage factors	Final stage factor(s)
Professional turnover model (Price & Mueller, 1981; Price, 1977)	Multistaged, causal, recursive model. Contains environmental, organizational, individual, and professional factors. Tested with 1,000 registered nurses in acute care agencies. Relationships are specified among factors for: Direction: causal +/- nature. Function: linear, probablistic	Opportunity. Routinization. Participation/decision making. Instrumental communication. Integration. Pay. Distributive justice. Promotional opportunity. Professionalism. General training. Kinship responsibility	Stage II. Job satisfaction. Stage III. Intent to stay	Actual, voluntary turnover
Professional autonomy and turnover model (Weisman, Alexander, & Chase, 1981)	Multistaged, causal, recursive model. Contains individual, professional, and organizational factors. Tested with 1,259 registered nurses in two university-affiliated hospitals. Relationships are specified among factors for: Direction: causal +/- nature. Function: linear probablistic	Personal attributes. Job-related attributes	Stage II. Autonomy. Stage III. Job satisfaction	Intent to leave. Turnover (voluntary)

Expectancy theory adapted to predict turnover (Vroom, 1964; Porter & Lawler, 1968; Seybolt, Pavett, & Walker, 1978)	Multistaged, causal, recursive model Contains individual factors Relationships are specified for: 　Direction: causal Studied 242 registered nurses and licensed practical nurses	Valence of outcomes Valence of performance Instrumentality	Stage II. Motivation 　Intervening factor: expectancy Stage III. Performance 　Intervening factors: ability, role perceptions Stage IV. Reward Stage V. Satisfaction 　Intervening factor: perceived equity 　　of reward	Actual, voluntary/involuntary turnover
Anticipated turnover model (Hinshaw & Atwood, 1982)	Multistaged, causal, recursive model Contains individual constructs Relationships are specified among constructs: 　Direction: causal 　　+/− nature 　Function: Linear Studied 140 registered nurses, licensed practical nurses, and nurses' aides in a university health sciences center	Expectation of tenure Mobility characteristics: age, education, pretenure	Stage II. Job stress Stage III. Job satisfaction Stage IV. Anticipated turnover	Actual turnover (voluntary and involuntary)

staff's potential termination. Study of these factors suggested that all three were strong mediators of prior staged factors, because they influenced actual voluntary and involuntary turnover (Hinshaw & Atwood, 1982; Price & Mueller, 1981; Weisman, Alexander, & Chase, 1981). The Anticipated Turnover Model contained a construct not evident in the other frameworks, i.e., job stress. Job stress was included because of the nursing profession's current concern with "burnout" as a factor in nonretention of professional nurses (Bailey, 1980; Bailey & Claus, Note 1).

Initial Stage Factors. A number of initial factors identified in the turnover models were predicted to impact indirectly on staff turnover. Certain characteristics of an individual influenced turnover: how mobile a nurse was in terms of family responsibility (Price & Mueller, 1981); age coupled with interest in settling down (Hinshaw & Atwood, 1982; Price, 1977; Seybolt et al., 1978); and initial expectations for staying in a position (Hinshaw & Atwood, 1982). Organizational characteristics such as leadership patterns (Alexander, Weisman, & Chase, 1982; Wolf, 1981); individual participation in decision making (Alexander et al., 1982; Price & Mueller, 1981; Weisman, Alexander, & Chase, 1981); integration, defined as the presence of close friends in an agency (Price & Mueller, 1981); and reward and pay incentives (Bowey, 1974; Lawler, 1971; McClosky, 1974; Wandelt, Pierce, & Widdowsen, 1981) were shown consistently to influence turnover. An environmental factor, job opportunity, defined as availability of other positions in a community, related positively to nursing staff turnover (Price & Mueller, 1981).

For the initial factors cited, the research findings showed that turnover was less apt to occur with increased participation in decision making, longer expectations of tenure at hire, presence of friends in the agency, increased colleague group cohesion, and higher pay. Individual staff who were younger and had fewer family responsibilities were more apt to terminate. In addition, the existence of multiple job opportunities in the community increased an individual's potential for turnover.

Midstage Factors. The midstage factors which consistently influenced turnover were performance rewards and incentives, job stress, role expectations and conflicts, job satisfaction, intent to stay (intent to leave), and anticipated turnover. The midstage factors tended to reflect individual staff responses or perceptions. Individual motivation interacted with ability and role perception to produce performance in the position which, if rewarded, would result in job satisfaction and retention in the agency (Porter & Lawler, 1968; Seybolt et al., 1978). Job stress (Atwood & Hinshaw, 1981; Consolvo, 1979) and role deprivation (Kramer, 1974;

Kramer & Baker, 1971) also influenced job satisfaction and, if high, increased turnover. In addition, the Weisman, Alexander, and Chase (1981) test of the Professional Autonomy Model suggested that autonomy was influenced by both personal and job-related attributes, and directly influenced job satisfaction but not turnover.

Job satisfaction was suggested to mediate the effect of the other midstage and initial stage factors on turnover (Gruneberg, 1976; Price & Mueller, 1981; Seybolt et al., 1978; Weisman, Alexander, & Chase, 1980). In the Price and Mueller (1981) study, eight factors influenced job satisfaction: opportunity, routinization, participation, instrumental communication, pay, promotional opportunity, general training, and kinship responsibility. One additional type of factor mediated the influence of job satisfaction on turnover: intent to stay or intent to leave (Price & Mueller, 1981; Weisman, Alexander, & Chase, 1981), which was defined as a dimension of organizational commitment (Porter & Lawler, 1968). The greater the intent to stay, the less turnover. Five factors influenced intent to stay: opportunity, job satisfaction, pay, general training, and kinship responsibility.

Turnover was influenced directly by opportunity, intent to stay, and general training. In the models, the explained variances for the final turnover stage were minimal, ranging from (R^2) .09 to .14 (Price & Mueller, 1981; Hinshaw & Atwood, 1982). In the Weisman, Alexander, and Chase (1981) study, job satisfaction significantly influenced intent to leave, which in turn influenced turnover but at similar low levels of explained variance. The anticipated turnover factor that also was staged between job satisfaction and turnover was meant to identify the individual's propensity for turnover (Hinshaw & Atwood, 1982; Seybolt et al., 1978). When the Anticipated Turnover Model was tested, mobility factors and job stress influenced anticipated turnover indirectly through job satisfaction. Anticipated turnover responses predicted actual turnover significantly (Hinshaw & Atwood, 1982), again with low explained variances.

The research linking job stress, satisfaction, and other factors to nursing staff turnover has several strengths. The Price and Mueller (1981) research on the Professional Turnover and Industrial Turnover models represented a program of research building on Price's 1977 synopsis of sociological and psychological studies in the field. The Weisman, Alexander, and Chase (1981) investigation extended the Price and Mueller (1981) work by the addition of the professional factor of autonomy. The Anticipated Turnover Model (Hinshaw & Atwood, 1982) illustrated a preventive approach to the field of turnover research. These studies, in addition to others cited, provided a solid description of the turnover phenomenon and factors that influenced it within acute care, metropolitan agencies. Similar evidence under other types of agency conditions (e.g., ambulatory clinics, long term care agencies, rural settings) was not so readily available.

The major weaknesses in the body of research on staff turnover were the low explained variances of the descriptive models; lack of replication of the studies except for the Price and Mueller (1981) and the Weisman, Alexander, and Chase (1981) research; and the different instruments used to measure the factors that made comparison across the studies difficult. In terms of the low explained variances for the models, questions must be asked about other factors not included in the models or about how measurement error could be masking certain factors and relationships.

Strategies for Decreasing Turnover

Numerous strategies targeted to decrease turnover were recommended. From their study of professional turnover, Price and Mueller (1981) suggested a series of interventions for reducing turnover. The difficulty was that, while reflecting their data, several of Price and Mueller's recommendations (e.g., recruit more diploma nurses) went counter to certain professional stances of nursing. Alexander, Weisman, and Chase (1982) recommended the use of various staffing patterns, workload levels, and primary nursing to increase job satisfaction and decrease terminations. All-registered-nurse staffing patterns have shown less turnover than mixed staffs (Hinshaw, Scofield, & Atwood, 1981). Increasing positive job experiences was suggested by Ullrich (1978) and Brief (1976), while support systems of formal colleague groups were recommended by Kramer (1974) and Kramer and Schmalenberg (1977). Bicultural training to merge professional and organizational orientations for new, graduate, registered nurses was suggested to result in a lower turnover rate (Holloran, Mishkin, & Hanson, 1980). Extensive employer intervention and discussion of reality versus expectation was recommended by Stryker-Gordon (1979) for decreasing turnover in nursing homes. Attitude surveys were used to provide information to administrators to sensitize both administrators and nursing staff to issues that led to turnover. Such strategies, for example, formal supervisory and colleague feedback sessions, facilitated the implementation of organizational interventions to decrease voluntary termination (Seybolt & Walker, 1980).

The major criticism of the research on strategies to decrease staff turnover was aimed at their lack of replication. In addition, many of the measures used in these studies did not cite psychometric properties. Future research with turnover factors should focus on evaluating interventions for promoting retention. However, few descriptive findings were available for guiding the choice of strategies with which to "retain" staff in agencies.

JOB STRESS

Investigators agreed that job stress involves disquieting influences, but differences occurred over whether stress was nonspecific, negative, or positive in value. Job stress was generally defined from Selye's (1976, p. 74) basic statement that "stress is a non-specific response of the body to any demand, whether it is caused by, or results in, pleasant or unpleasant conditions." Job stress involves those demands encountered within the roles and functions of employment. The stress response was described as both biological and psychological in nature. While Selye (1976) suggested that stress is neither negative nor positive in value but nonspecific, other investigators disputed this stance (Lazarus, Cohen, & Folkman, 1980; Mason, 1971). Lazarus et al. (1980) and Broverman and Lazarus (1958) suggested that stress takes on a positive or negative value depending on the responder's perception. The stress was suggested to be cognitively mediated and thus assigned the value (Bailey, 1980; Broverman & Lazarus, 1958; Cleland, 1965).

The Yerkes-Dodson Law (Benson & Allen, 1980; Cleland, 1965) as related to professional job stress suggested that very high or low levels of stress decreased individual productivity. Bailey (1980) dealt with factors that generated job stress for intensive-care-unit (ICU) nurses, suggesting that consequences of extremely high job stress could be "burnout" (Bailey, 1980; Stehle, 1981). "Burnout" is a term used to describe nurses who have "depleted or exhausted their emotional and physical energies in dealing with the stressors of the work environment" (McConnell, 1979, p. 5).

The relationship of extreme job stress to productivity and turnover may not be direct. Early research tracing the relationship of job stress to turnover or loss of productive individuals suggested that job stress was mediated by job satisfaction (Hinshaw & Atwood, 1982). For future study, many questions remain: What is the relationship of job stress to staff productivity and retention? Does the relationship of job stress to staff productivity and retention vary across clinical services *or* according to a professional's socialization pattern *or* according to individual characteristics such as locus of control?

Influential Factors

Factors suggested as influencing job stress usually were defined as types of stressors (i.e., sources of stress) that affect or influence response (e.g., Bailey, Steffen, & Grout, 1980; Gentry, Foster, & Froehling, 1972; Magill, 1982; Stehle, 1981). The categories of stressors generated from multiple sources were given as: the physical work environment (Bailey, Steffen, & Grout, 1980); professional-bureaucratic role conflict (Kramer, 1974; Kramer & Baker, 1971; Kramer & Schmalenberg, 1977); role strain and tension from multiple expectations (Brosnan & Johnston, 1980; Cleland, 1965; Hinshaw & Oakes, 1977; Magill, 1982); management, communication patterns, and leadership style with nursing administration (Bailey, Steffen, & Grout, 1980; Benson & Allen, 1980; Huckabay & Jagla, 1979); staffing and workload problems (Anderson & Basteyns, 1981; Atwood & Hinshaw, 1981; Bailey, Steffen, & Grout, 1980); negative patient outcomes (Anderson & Basteyns, 1981; Grout, Steffen, & Bailey, 1981); communications with physicians (Huckabay & Jagla, 1979); lack of participation in policy and practice decisions (Magill, 1982); and inadequate knowledge and skills for role functions (Bailey, Steffen, & Grout, 1980; Huckabay & Jagla, 1979). These numerous factors were prioritized differently in various reports.

Stress and burnout were studied extensively for nurses functioning in intensive care units, (e.g., Anderson & Basteyns, 1981; Bailey, Steffen, & Grout, 1980; Huckabay & Jagla, 1979; McConnell, 1979). Less extensively studied was stress experienced by general unit staff, ambulatory care staff, or others (Brosnan & Johnston, 1980; Cleland, 1965). Still less information was available on types of stress experienced by nurses across clinical services.

Strategies for Handling Job Stress

A number of individual and organization strategies were described in the literature for coping with or adapting to job stress. Few evaluations were found of the effectiveness of the strategies in terms of nursing staff performance, productivity, and client outcomes. Individual stress reduction strategies included exercise (Zindler-Wernert & Bailey, 1980) and relaxation programs (e.g., Benson & Allen, 1980; Neal & Cooper, 1980); assertiveness training (Neal & Cooper, 1980); imagery strategies (Neal & Cooper, 1980); and understanding and obtaining a commitment to one's self (Kobasa, 1979; Magill, 1982).

Organizational strategies for stress reduction were programs planned by employers specific to certain identified job stressors. For example, Stanford University's stress management program for ICU nurses was based on the factors identified in prior study (Bailey, Walker, & Madsen, 1980). Certain stress reduction strategies were matched with the types of stressors experienced by the staff (Bailey, Walker, & Madsen, 1980). A number of organizations used support groups to help staff handle stress (e.g., Scully, 1981) or combined inservice education/support teams (e.g., Stillman & Strasser, 1980). Changing staffing patterns, shifting workloads, and negotiating staff assignments were other mechanisms for varying or decreasing job stress (Alexander, Weisman, & Chase, 1981; McConnell, 1979).

Several future trends were evident for systematically and creatively identifying strategies that will decrease or allow staff to cope with job stress. Grout et al. (1981) and Hinshaw and Atwood (1982) suggested that the "satisfiers" in an employment setting can be used to offset the stressors. Magill (1982) recommended that studies be focused on the "brightly burning" staff instead of the burnouts. From descriptions of those who were coping well with job stress and remaining in the employment system, information could be obtained for helping others to use such successful coping strategies. In addition, organizations may identify structural and environmental strategies (e.g., primary nursing) that can be used to keep staff "brightly burning" (Alexander et al., 1981; Magill, 1982).

JOB SATISFACTION

Traditional Versus Nontraditional Definitions

Several conceptual definitions for job satisfaction were supported empirically (Price, 1972), but two issues persist: unidimensional versus multidimensional concept, and the continuum of job satisfaction to dissatisfaction versus the continuum of satisfaction to no satisfaction. In the traditional unidimensional definition of job satisfaction used in macrosociological research, the worker balanced various satisfaction factors into a summary response (Kahn, Wolfe, Quinn, & Snoek, 1964; Kalleberg, 1977). Job satisfaction was comprised of persistent feelings by the worker toward specific, identifiable aspects of the job (Smith, Kendall, & Hulin, 1969; Note 2.)

The Herzberg (1968) Two Factor Theory definition countered the traditional one. Job satisfaction was not the opposite of job dissatisfaction, but rather each ranged from none to a lot. Herzberg's two factors included potential satisfiers (e.g., motivators) and hygiene factors (e.g., pay), which contributed differentially to dissatisfaction (Everly & Falcione, 1976; Longest, 1974; Palola & Larson, 1965; Slavitt, Stamps, Piedmont, & Haase, 1978).

Operational definitions were indexed primarily by rating scales, many of which had unspecified validity and reliability. However, when psychometric assessments were cited, they met minimum criteria (e.g., alpha for immature scales = .70, per Nunnally, 1978). Even though most scales were originally used in private industry, they were considered in this review only if also used in nursing research, for the key issues are psychometric testing and development of indices specifically for job satisfaction in professional nursing and health care settings.

In addition, because satisfaction levels differed considerably for specified factors, a multifactor scale versus a summed total was required for sensitive measurement and for guiding intervention. For example, Longest (1974) reported marked differences in the satisfiers identified by registered nurses in medium-sized general community hospitals in contrast to industrial workers. Hurka (1972) found that short range satisfiers were more important to registered nurses than long range ones, possibly because few long range ones, such as opportunities for advancement, were available.

The Brayfield and Rothe (1951) 18-item Likert-type job satisfaction scale, devised for study of industrial workers' attitudes, was used in some health care settings (Alexander et al., 1981; Brosnan & Johnston, 1980). Psychometric estimates with nonprofessonal workers have been made (Price, 1972). Atwood and Hinshaw (1980) adapted the Brayfield and Rothe (1951) scale for use with inpatient and outpatient nursing. The new scale, which was tested psychometrically, indexed satisfaction with job enjoyment, quality of care, care/comfort measures given, job interest, and time to do the job. The tested Index of Work Satisfaction (Slavitt, Stamps, Piedmont, & Haase, 1978, 1979; Stamps, Piedmont, Slavitt, & Haase, 1978) contained six Likert-type subscales (pay, autonomy, task requirements, organizational requirements, interaction, and job status/prestige). Munson and Heda (1974) modified the Porter and Lawler (1968) quantified interview scale to index job satisfaction among hospital nursing staff. The resultant tested rating scale indexed involvement, interpersonal, intrinsic, and extrinsic satisfaction. As a consideration for future research, since multiple subscales of job satisfaction provide a choice of which aspects to measure, investigators need to predict which aspects will change as a result of their interventions and select indices to measure those specific aspects.

Influential Factors and Strategies for Enhancing Job Satisfaction

In health care settings, primarily descriptive studies, with widely ranging, predominantly convenience samples, were reported for community health nurses (Koerner, 1981), hospital inpatient general and ICU staff (Duxbury & Armstrong, 1982; Munson & Heda, 1974; Ullrich, 1978; Weisman, Dear, Alexander, & Chase, 1981), outpatient staff (Berkowitz & Bennis, 1961), and nursing faculty (Bauder, 1982; Grandjean, Bonjean, & Aiken, 1982). Job satisfaction among staff (nonprofessionals and office workers) in various positions also was studied (Bullough, 1974).

Research results did not convey consensus regarding a single, most predictive theoretical model, and industrial studies have untested generalizability to health care workers. However, several conceptualizations are considered here. According to Ewen, Smith, Hulin, and Locke (1966), some satisfiers were more powerful than others in influencing job satisfaction. The satisfier/dissatisfier dichotomy may not be predictive (House & Wignor, 1967), and a net satisfaction effect may be estimated by satisfiers minus dissatisfiers. Future intervention strategies could include maximizing that sum or ratio. In Herzberg's Two Factor Theory (Herzberg, Mausner, & Snyderman, 1959) of industrial work motivation, the factors intrinsic to the work, such as responsibility, formed the satisfaction-no satisfaction continuum, whereas the extrinsic ones, such as company policy, likely formed the dissatisfaction-no dissatisfaction continuum (Herzberg, 1968). Most of the factors are controllable. In his analysis of five interpretations of the Herzberg theory based on case studies in multiple industrial groups, King (1970) corroborated the Ewen, Smith, Hulin, and Locke (1966) work by concluding that satisfaction was enhanced more by the combined intrinsic motivators than dissatisfaction was influenced by extrinsic hygiene factors. In his descriptive study of a volunteer sample of 40 private general hospital nurses, Ullrich (1978) indicated that some of the intrinsic factors were dissatisfiers. Turnover was increased by dissatisfiers.

In contrast to the Herzberg Two Factor Theory, job satisfaction and dissatisfaction were on a continuum in the Hulin and Smith linear model (1964); that is, the opposite of satisfaction was dissatisfaction. The relationship between role tension or stress and job satisfaction was described for the Hirschowitz (1974; Brosnan & Johnston, 1980) stages of the change process. March and Simon (1958) proposed that higher expectation of reward is correlated with job satisfaction and that high level of aspiration is associated with low satisfaction. Individual satisfaction may be related indirectly to group productivity. Job satisfaction buffered the effects of job stress in turnover (Hinshaw & Atwood, 1980).

Historically, clear identification has been hampered by marginal validity and reliability of measures (Evans, 1969; Kalleberg, 1974). Compendia of empirical findings ranging widely in quality at the macrosociological level included general industrial studies (e.g., Gruneberg, 1976; Porter & Steers, 1973) and health care industry research (e.g., Georgopoulos, 1975; Robinson & Connors, 1960). Several studies with large sample sizes yielded factors contributing to various aspects of primarily industrial job satisfaction (Kalleberg 1977; Kalleberg & Griffin, 1980; Kuhlen, 1963; Orpen, 1979; Perry, 1978; Schaffer, 1954; Tatro, 1974). Statistically significant factors included organizational features, job characteristics, rewards, opportunities for meeting needs, specialization, age, and occupation. Key factors influencing job satisfaction in multiple settings included age (Anderson & Haag, 1963; Hoppcock, 1935; Slavitt et al., 1979), sex (Hulin & Smith, 1964), intelligence (Hulin & Smith, 1964), education (Slavitt et al., 1979), experience as a nurse (Slavitt et al., 1979; Weisman, Dear, Alexander, & Chase, 1981), tenure (Hulin & Smith, 1964), and position in the hierarchy (Anderson & Haag, 1963; Munson & Heda, 1974; Slavitt et al., 1979). Significant health care environment factors included the clinical service and type of unit (Brosnan & Johnston, 1980; Slavitt et al., 1979), nursing care delivery model (Alexander et al., 1981; Hinshaw et al., 1981), degree of professionalization and organizational climate (Bauder, 1982; Duxbury & Armstrong, 1982; Grandjean et al., 1982; Tatro, 1974), supervision, and interpersonal relationships (Berkowitz & Bennis, 1961; Herzberg et al., 1959; Hoppcock, 1935; Smith et al., 1969).

Characteristics of the job itself included status (Herzberg et al., 1959; Hoppcock, 1935; Koerner, 1981), autonomy (Donovan, 1980; Grandjean et al., 1982; Marriner & Craigie, 1977; McClosky, 1974), repetitiveness (Vroom, 1964; Smith, Kendall, & Hulin, Note 2), tasks (Bullough, 1974;

Ullrich, 1978), job outcomes (Munson & Heda, 1974), and pay (Kalleberg, 1977; Lerch, 1982; Slavitt et al., 1978).

A serious issue for future consideration is that the suggested influencing factors were legion, often applied conditionally, and had been tested only one or two at a time by different investigators in single studies rather than in programs of research. Thus, the relative impact of the variables, acting simultaneously and conditionally, is unknown.

Job satisfaction research in nursing contains alternate conceptual definitions and models, inherited primarily from organizational sociology. Nursing research to date shows some adaptation and extension of earlier work, with the heaviest emphasis in the validity and reliability areas. Almost all research cited is descriptive in design, uses an unspecified or convenience sample ranging from 32 to 1496, and is based on limited populations. Generalizability is problematic.

SUMMARY, RESEARCH DIRECTIONS

Researchers in the field of nursing turnover, job stress, and job satisfaction have been prolific, with much of the knowledge contributed by organizational sociologists and psychologists. While these contributions have been extremely valuable, a number of avenues for future research become evident.

The majority of the investigations on nursing turnover, job stress, and job satisfaction contained factors influencing each, their impact on other factors, and the staged processes delineating the direct and indirect relationships of numerous factors to ultimate staff turnover. Less research evidence was available on the effectiveness and efficiency of strategies for handling stress, increasing satisfaction, and retaining staff. Much of the literature is theoretical in nature, advancing substantive recommendations without presenting data to evaluate nursing staff, cost, or client outcomes. Such an evaluation process is crucial for a practice profession that needs not only to identify factors that influence the delivery of care but is also accountable for manipulating those factors and instituting strategies to counter negative consequences, e.g., high voluntary staff turnover.

Instituting programs of research in these fields will be a complex endeavor. Present investigators suggest that factors that influence turnover, job stress, and satisfaction are conditional. Consequences and strategies for dealing with these factors vary by individual characteristics, organization-al-structural entities, and types of clinical service. Systematic, careful manipulation and testing of numerous subsets of these conditions are required.

In addition, knowledge adapted from other disciplines based on industrial organizations and nonprofessional workers requires testing before the findings can be generalized to primarily professional staff functioning in service-oriented institutions. These investigations have been started. More attention should be focused on the addition of professional factors, such as the impact of control over nursing practice and professional autonomy on staff stress, job satisfaction, and turnover; Weisman, Alexander, and Chase (1981) initiated such research. The inclusion of professional factors in the studies may enhance the explained variances.

Both conceptual and methodological problems ensue when measurement difficulties occur. Kalleberg (1974) suggested that part of the problem in obtaining higher explained variances and identifying factors influencing job stress, satisfaction, and turnover traditionally has been the measurement instruments used in the investigations. Many factors that influence or were consequences of staff turnover, stress, or satisfaction may not have been documented systematically because of instability in the measures and lack of validity information.

Several methodological issues transcend nursing turnover, job stress, and job satisfaction. The first is generalizability, a concern of managers and researchers alike. Sample sizes for the empirical research on job satisfaction ranged widely; for example, $n = 22$ to 557 in the job satisfaction citations. In addition, few of the samples were selected randomly. Further, most of the studies have yet to be replicated. Another methodological issue is reliance on descriptive designs. A positive trend is the increasing emphasis on causal or predictive models for understanding the prevention of job stress, dissatisfaction, and turnover versus the ex post facto studies more prevalent historically. A notable challenge is finding available field settings and access to the sample sizes required for sensitivity to various kinds of health care workers and for supporting statistical tests of intervention models.

A higher percentage of research efforts in staff turnover, stress, and satisfaction should be concentrated on programs of research. The programs should include formulating and testing innovative intervention strategies; evaluating the impact of interventions on staff, clients, and costs; and testing the degree to which solutions posed in other industrial settings apply to the health care industry.

REFERENCE NOTES

1. Bailey, J. T., & Claus, K. *Summary of a study of stress in intensive care nursing in northern California*. San Francisco: University of California School of Nursing, Fall–Winter, 1977–78.
2. Smith, P. C., Kendall, L. M., & Hulin, C. L. *Cornell studies of job satisfaction: I–VI*. Ithaca, N.Y.: Cornell University, 1969.

REFERENCES

Alexander, C. S., Weisman, C. S., & Chase, G. A. Evaluating primary nursing in hospitals: Examination of effects on nursing staff. *Medical Care*, 1981, *19*, 80–89.

Alexander, C. S., Weisman, C. S., & Chase, G. A. Determinants of staff nurses' perceptions of autonomy within different clinical contexts. *Nursing Research*, 1982, *31*, 48–52.

Anderson, C. A., & Basteyns, M. Stress and the critical care nurse reaffirmed. *Journal of Nursing Administration*, 1981, *11*(1), 31–34.

Anderson, W., & Haag, G. A study of hospital employee attitudes. *Hospital Management*, 1963, *96*(1), 38–41.

Atwood, J. R., & Hinshaw, A. S. Job satisfaction instrument: A program of development and testing. In *Communicating nursing research*, (Vol. 12). Boulder, Colo.: Western Interstate Commission on Higher Education, 1980. (Abstract)

Atwood, J. R., & Hinshaw, A. S. Job stress instrument development program. *Western Journal of Research in Nursing*, 1981, *3*, 48. (Abstract)

Bailey, J. T. Stress and stress management: An overview. *Journal of Nursing Education*, 1980, *19*(6), 5–8.

Bailey, J. T., Steffen, S. M., & Grout, J. W. The stress audit: Identifying the stressors of ICU nursing. *Journal of Nursing Education*, 1980 *19*(6), 15–25.

Bailey, J. T., Walker, D., & Madsen, N. The design of a stress management program for Stanford intensive care nurses. *Journal of Nursing Education*, 1980, *19*(6), 26–30.

Bauder, L. Discontent and crisis at schools of nursing: The consequences of unmet human needs. *Western Journal of Nursing Research*, 1982, *4*, 35–48.

Benson, H., & Allen, R. L. How much stress is too much? *Harvard Business Review*, 1980, *58*(5), 86–92.

Berkowitz, N. H., & Bennis, W. G. Interaction patterns in formal service-oriented organizations. *Administrative Science Quarterly*, 1961, *6*, 25–50.

Bowey, A. M. *A guide to manpower planning*. London: Macmillan, 1974.

Brayfield, A. H., & Rothe, H. F. An index of job satisfaction. *Journal of Applied Psychology*, 1951, *35*, 307–311.

Brief, A. P. Turnover among hospital nurses: A suggested model. *Journal of Nursing Administration*, 1976, *6*(8), 55–58.

Brosnan, J., & Johnston, M. Stressed but satisfied: Organizational change in ambulatory care. *Journal of Nursing Administration*, 1980, *10*(11), 43–46.

Broverman, D. M., & Lazarus, R. S. Individual differences in task performance under conditions of cognitive interference. *Journal of Personality*, 1958, *26*, 94–105.

Bullough, B. Is the nurse practitioner role a source of increased work satisfaction? *Nursing Research*, 1974, *23*, 183; 193.

Cleland, V. S. The effect of stress on performance. *Nursing Research*, 1965, *14*, 292–298.

Consolvo, C. A. Nurse turnover in the newborn intensive care unit. *Journal of Gynecological Nursing*, 1979, *8*, 201–204.

Donovan, L. What nurses want (and what they're getting). *RN Magazine*, 1980, *43*(4), 22–30.

Duxbury, M. L., & Armstrong, G. D. Calculating nurse turnover indices. *Journal of Nursing Administration*, 1982, *12*(3), 18–24.

Evans, M. G. Conceptual and operational problems in the measurement of various aspects of job satisfaction. *Journal of Applied Psychology*, 1969, *53* (Part I), 93–101.

Everly, G., & Falcione, R. Perceived dimensions of job satisfaction for staff registered nurses. *Nursing Research*, 1976, *25*, 346–348.

Ewen, R. B., Smith, P. C., Hulin, C. L., & Locke, E. A. An empirical test of the Herzberg two factor theory. *Journal of Applied Psychology*, 1966, *50*, 544–550.

Gentry, W. D., Foster, S. B., & Froehling, S. Psychological response to situational stress in intensive and nonintensive nursing. *Heart & Lung*, 1972, *1*, 793–796.

Georgopoulos, B. (Ed.). *Hospital organization research: Review and source book*. Philadelphia: Saunders, 1975.

Grandjean, B. D., Bonjean, C. M., & Aiken, L. H. The effect of centralized decision-making on work satisfaction among nursing educators. *Research in Nursing and Health*, 1982, *5*, 29–36.

Grout, J. W., Steffen, S. M., & Bailey, J. T. The stresses and the satisfiers of the intensive care unit: A survey. *Critical Care Quarterly*, 1981, *3*(4), 35–45.

Gruneberg, M. M. (Ed.). *Job satisfaction*. New York: Wiley, 1976.

Herzberg, F. I. One more time: How do you motivate employees? *Harvard Business Review*, 1968, *46*(1), 53–62.

Herzberg, F., Mausner, B., & Snyderman, B. *The motivation to work*. New York: Wiley, 1959.

Hinshaw, A. S., & Atwood, J. R. Anticipated turnover: A pilot instrument. In M. V. Batey (Ed.), *Communicating nursing research* (Vol. 12). Boulder, Colo.: Western Interstate Commission on Higher Education, 1980. (Abstract)

Hinshaw, A. S., & Atwood, J. R. Anticipated turnover: A preventive approach. *Western Journal of Nursing Research*, 1982, *4*, 54–55.

Hinshaw, A. S., & Oakes, D. Theoretical model testing: Patients', nurses', and physicians' expectations of quality nursing care. In M. V. Batey (Ed.), *Communicating nursing research* (Vol. 10). Boulder, Colo.: Western Interstate Commission on Higher Education, 1977.

Hinshaw, A. S., Scofield, R., & Atwood, J. R. Staff, patient and cost outcomes of all-registered-nurse staffing. *Journal of Nursing Administration,* 1981, *11*(11 & 12), 30–36.

Hirschowitz, R. G. The human aspects of managing transition. *Personnel,* 1974, *50,* 8–17.

Holloran, S. D., Mishkin, B. H., & Hanson, B. L. Bicultural training for new graduates. *Journal of Nursing Administration,* 1980, *10*(2), 17–24.

Hoppcock, R. *Job satisfaction.* New York: Harper, 1935.

House, R. J., & Wignor, L. A. Herzberg's dual-factor theory of job satisfaction and motivation: A review of the evidence and criticism. *Personnel Psychology,* 1967, *20,* 369–389.

Huckabay, L. M. D., & Jagla, B. Nurses' stress factors in the intensive care unit. *Journal of Nursing Administration,* 1979, *9*(2), 21–26.

Hulin, C. L., & Smith, P. C. Sex differences in job satisfaction. *Journal of Applied Psychology,* 1964, *48,* 88–92.

Hurka, J. J. Career orientations of registered nurses working in hospitals. *Hospital Administration,* 1972, *17*(1), 26.

Kahn, R. L., Wolfe, D. M., Quinn, R. P., & Snoek, J. D. *Organizational stress: Studies in role conflict and ambiguity.* New York: Wiley, 1964.

Kahne, M. J. Suicides in mental hospitals: A study of the effects of personnel and patient turnover. *Journal of Health & Social Behavior,* 1968, *9,* 255–266.

Kalleberg, A. L. A causal approach to the measurement of job satisfaction. *Social Science Research,* 1974, *3,* 299–322.

Kalleberg, A. L. Work values and job rewards: A theory of job satisfaction. *American Sociological Review,* 1977, *42,* 124–143.

Kalleberg, A. L., & Griffin, L. J. Class, operation and inequality in job rewards. *American Journal of Sociology,* 1980, *85,* 731–768.

King, N. Clarification and evaluation of the two-factor theory of job satisfaction. *Psychological Bulletin,* 1970, *74,* 18–31.

Kobasa, S. C. Stressful life events, personality, and health: An inquiry into hardiness. *Journal of Personality and Social Psychology,* 1979, *34,* 1–11.

Koerner, B. L. Selected correlates of job performance of community health nurses. *Nursing Research,* 1981, *30,* 43–48.

Kramer, M. *Reality shock.* St. Louis: Mosby, 1974.

Kramer, M., & Baker, C. The exodus: Can we prevent it? *Journal of Nursing Administration,* 1971, *1*(3), 15–30.

Kramer, M., & Schmalenberg, C. *Path to biculturalism.* Wakefield, Mass.: Nursing Resources, 1977.

Kuhlen, R. G. Needs, perceived need satisfaction opportunities, and satisfaction with occupation. *Journal of Applied Psychology,* 1963, *47,* 56–64.

Lawler, E. E. *Pay and organizational effectiveness.* New York: McGraw-Hill, 1971.

Lazarus, R. S., Cohen, J. B., & Folkman, S. Psychological stress and adaptation: Some unresolved issues. In H. Selye (Ed.), *Selye's guide to stress research* (Vol. 1). New York: Van Nostrand Reinhold, 1980.

Lerch, E. M. Criteria-based performance appraisals. *Nursing Management,* 1982, *13*(7), 28–31.

Longest, B. B., Jr. Job satisfaction for registered nurses in the hospital setting. *Journal of Nursing Administration*, 1974, *4*(3), 46–52.

Magill, K. A. Burnin, burnout and the brightly burning. *Nursing Management*, 1982, *13*(7), 17–21.

March, J. G., & Simon, H. A. *Organizations*. New York: Wiley, 1958.

Marriner, A., & Craigie, D. Job satisfaction and mobility of nursing educators in baccalaureate and higher degree programs in the west. *Nursing Research*, 1977, *26*, 349–360.

Mason, J. W. A re-evaluation of the concept of "non-specificity" in stress theory. *Journal of Psychiatric Research*, 1971, *8*, 323–333.

McClosky, J. Influence of rewards and incentives on staff nurse turnover rate. *Nursing Research*, 1974, *23*, 238–247.

McConnell, E. Burnout and the critical care nurse. *Critical Care Update*, 1979, *6*, 5–14.

Mobley, W. H., Griffeth, R. W., Hand, H. H., & Meglino, B. M. Review and conceptual analysis of the employee turnover process. *Psychological Bulletin*, 1979, *86*, 493–522.

Munson, F. C., & Heda, S. S. An instrument for measuring nursing satisfaction. *Nursing Research*, 1974, *23*, 159–166.

Neal, M., & Cooper, P. Diagnosing stress in your nursing world. *CE Focus*, 1980, *3*(1), 5–12.

Nunnally, J. *Psychometric theory*. New York: McGraw-Hill, 1978.

Orpen, C. The effects of job enrichment on employee satisfaction, motivation, involvement and performance: A field experiment. *Human Relations*, 1979, *32*, 189–217.

Palola, E. G., & Larson, W. R. Some dimensions of job satisfaction among hospital personnel. *Social Science Research*, 1965, *49*, 201–213.

Perry, H. B., III. The job satisfaction of physician assistants: A causal analysis. *Social Science and Medicine*, 1978, *12*, 377–385.

Porter, L. W., & Lawler, E. E., III. *Managerial attitudes and performances*. Homewood, Ill.: Irvine, 1968.

Porter, L. W., & Steers, R. M. Organizational, work and personal factors in employee turnover and absenteeism. *Psychological Bulletin*, 1973, *80*, 151–176.

Price, J. L. *Handbook of organizational measurement*. Lexington, Mass,: Heath, 1972.

Price, J. L. *The study of turnover*. Ames, Iowa: Iowa State University Press, 1977.

Price, J. L., & Mueller, C. W. *Professional turnover: The cases of nurses*. New York: Medical & Scientific Books, 1981.

Revans, R. W. *Standards of morale*. London: Oxgord, 1964.

Robinson, H. A., & Connors, R. P. Job satisfaction research of 1959. *Personnel Guidance Journal*, 1960, *39*, 47–52.

Schaffer, R. H. Job satisfaction as related to need satisfaction in work. *Psychological Monographs*, 1954, *67*(14, Whole No. 364), 1–29.

Scully, R. Staff support groups: Helping nurses to help themselves. *Journal of Nursing Administration*, 1981, *11*(3), 48–51.

Selye, H. *Stress in health and disease*. Boston: Butterworth, 1976.

Seybolt, J. W., Pavett, C., & Walker, D. D. Turnover among nurses: It can be managed. *Journal of Nursing Administration*, 1978, *8*(9), 4–9.

Seybolt, J. W., & Walker, D. D. Attitude survey proves to be a powerful tool for reversing turnover. *Hospitals*, 1980, *54*(9), 77–80.

Slavitt, D. B., Stamps, P. L., Piedmont, E. B., & Haase, A. M. Nurses' satisfaction with their work situation. *Nursing Research*, 1978, *27*, 114–120.

Slavitt, D. B., Stamps, P. L., Piedmont, E. B., & Haase, A. M. Measuring nurses' job satisfaction. *Hospital and Health Services Administration*, 1979, *24*(3), 62–76.

Smith, P. C., Kendall, L. M., & Hulin, C. L. *The measurement of satisfaction in work and retirement: A strategy for the study of attitudes.* Chicago: Rand McNally, 1969.

Stamps, P. L., Piedmont, E. B., Slavitt, D. B., & Haase, A. M. Measurement of work satisfaction among health professionals. *Medical Care*, 1978, *16*, 337–352.

Stehle, J. L. Critical care nursing stress: The findings revisited. *Nursing Research*, 1981, *30*, 182–186.

Stillman, S. M., & Strasser, B. L. Helping critical care nurses with work-related stress. *Journal of Nursing Administration*, 1980, *10*(1), 28–31.

Stryker-Gordon, R. Minnesota study suggests means of reducing turnover rates in nursing homes. *Journal of Nursing Administration*, 1979, *9*(4), 17–20.

Tatro, E. H. Professional organizational climate and job satisfaction of nurses employed in hospitals (Doctoral dissertation, University of Illinois at Urbana-Champaign, 1974). *Dissertation Abstracts International*, 1974, *35*, 5500B. (University Microfilms No. 75–11, 678)

Ullrich, R. A. Herzberg revisited: Factors in job dissatisfaction. *Journal of Nursing Administration*, 1978, *8*(10), 19–24.

Vroom, V. H. *Work and motivation.* New York: Wiley, 1964.

Wandelt, M., Pierce, P., & Widdowsen, R. Why nurses leave nursing and what can be done about it. *American Journal of Nursing*, 1981, *81*, 72–77.

Weisman, C. S., Alexander, C. S., & Chase, G. A. Job satisfaction among hospital nurses: A longitudinal study. *Health Services Research*, 1980, *15*, 341–346.

Weisman, C. S., Alexander, C. S., & Chase, G. A. Determinants of hospital staff nurse turnover. *Medical Care*, 1981, *19*, 431–443.

Weisman, C. S., Dear, M. R., Alexander, C. S., & Chase, G. A. Employment patterns among newly hired hospital staff nurses: Comparison of nursing graduates and experienced nurses. *Nursing Research*, 1981, *30*, 188–191.

Wolf, G. A. Nursing turnover: Some causes and solutions. *Nursing Outlook*, 1981, *29*, 233–236.

Zindler-Wernert, P., & Bailey, J. T. Coping with stress through an "on-site" running program for Stanford ICU nurses. *Journal of Nursing Education*, 1980, *19*(6), 34–37.

CHAPTER 7

Interorganizational Relations Research in Nursing Care Delivery Systems

Janelle C. Krueger

School of Nursing

University of Colorado Health Sciences Center

CONTENTS

The focus of this review is on research related to the interaction of organizations with one another or their environment and with the contribution of this interorganizational relations (IOR) research to the understanding of the structure and decision making in organizations. A general introduction to the field seemed necessary because of both the sparsity and the great need for such research in nursing. A few studies related to nursing are included. Suggestions for future directions in IOR research in nursing appear in the summary.

The study of organizations can be categorized into three general types: structural, social psychological, and ecological. Investigators using structural and social psychological frameworks, referred to as intraorganizational research, seek to identify factors related to improving the efficiency or performance within an organization. Early organizational and management research and theory emphasized the ways that the technology, or the means for getting the work done, should be structured to maximize efficiency and economic return (Gulick & Urwich, 1937; Taylor, 1911; Weber, 1924/1947). The serendipitous finding of the Hawthorne effect (Mayo, 1945; Roethlisberger & Dickson, 1940), which implied that worker productivity was influenced as much by feelings and sentiments as by rational economic factors, opened a whole new field of organizational analysis. The social psychological level of study focused on the importance of the informal organization, a part of the internal environment (March & Simon, 1958; Porter, Lawler, & Hackman, 1975).

In both structural and social psychological research, the organization was viewed as a closed system. Although approximately 90 % of organizational research efforts have focused on the internal system and the development of individual action theories, only about 10 % of the variance in organizational performance is attributed to the administrators' actions (Lieberson & O'Connor, 1972; Salancik & Pfeffer, 1977). Even though Weber's (1924/1947) description of bureaucracy was developed from his comparative studies of the effect of social structure on organizations, only in the past 30 years have a few sociologists (Bendix, 1956; Parsons, 1960; Selznick, 1949, 1957), economists (Philips, 1960; Scherer, 1970; Stigler, 1968), or anthropologists (Sahlins & Service, 1960; White, 1949) begun to include the relationship between the environment and the organization in their research. When researchers began to study the organization as an open system, they described survival or adaptation to a changing environment as the central problem of the organization.

EARLY INTERORGANIZATIONAL EFFORTS

The conceptual framework for IOR research grew out of formulations of Lewin (1935/1955) and Parsons (1937, 1951) that related to human action at the level of the individual. These writers viewed human action as the product of the interaction of the individual's aspirations, standards, and knowledge or belief about causation, as well as the presenting situations, opportunties, and constraints. The individual searched within himself and the environment for opportunities in harmony with his aspirations, constraints, and values.

In later writings, Parsons, a student of Weber, developed his general analytical systems model that included the individual as well as collectivities, from small primary groups to entire societies (Parsons, Bales, & Shils, 1953). Parsons believed that every social system must satisfy four basic needs, which he identified by the acronym AGIL. Adaptation was the problem of acquiring sufficient resources, while Goal attainment included the setting and implementation of goals. Integration referred to maintaining solidarity or coordination among the subunits of the system. Latency or pattern maintenance was concerned with creating, preserving, and transmitting the system's distinctive culture and values. Linkages and interactions among and between all parts of the system and its environment were central to the schema of Parsons et al. (1953).

The theoretical notions of Parsons were given empirical credence by Dill (1958), who used the term "task environment" to describe parts of the environment that he found relevant to setting and attaining organizational goals. In a study of Norwegian firms, he identified four task environment sections: customers; suppliers of materials, labor, capital, equipment, and work space; competitors for both markets and resources; and regulatory groups, including governmental agencies, unions, and interfirm associations.

The belief of Parsons et al. (1953) that all organizations served some societal function or need was supported by Levine and White (1961). In their study of relationships among community health agencies, they defined "domain" as the field staked out by an organization in terms of diseases covered, population served, and services rendered. Attaining a viable domain is a critical political problem for any profession. For example, nursing is currently struggling to define its domain. The struggle will intensify as the competition for clients becomes more intense.

In 1967 Thompson pulled together a conceptual inventory on the behavior of organizations that was based on Parsons's ideas. He considered organizations as actors operating in an open system interdependent with their environment. He developed propositions dealing with buffering environmental influences; defending domains; designing technology and structure; boundary-spanning activities; assessing organizations; and exercising discretion and control. Thompson characterized external and internal uncertainty as the fundamental problems for organizations. His plea was that organizations be studied in relation to their environment.

The focus on the field of IOR as a field of analysis began with Evan (1966), Guetzkow (1966), Thompson (1967), and Turk (1971). Over the years, many conceptual frameworks were offered, but none received wide acceptance or adequate empirical validation. Some provided useful insights, but none had dependable predictive power.

An underlying premise was that an interorganizational relationship has the same properties as any organized collective behavior. That is, behavior is goal-directed, members are interdependent, and the relationship can be treated as a unit in terms of process, structure, and outcome (Van de Ven & Ferry, 1980). Acceptance of the premise that the organization is an appropriate unit of analysis led to the development of at least four major categories of IOR studies. These categories and their subdivisions have been summarized below as situational factors, structure, process, and outcome.

Situational Factors

Once formed, organizations have a propensity for self-maintaining behavior; the ultimate desired outcome is survival. Since no organization has all the resources necessary to survive, the formation of relationships with others is inevitable. In forming links, organizations strive to maintain their autonomy or capability to select the course of action or strategy most favorable to them (Van de Ven & Ferry, 1980). They only form relationships with others to fulfill a strong internal need for resources belonging to another organization or agency. This resource dependence viewpoint stressed the active role played by organizations in adapting to their changing environment. Two versions of this approach are the political economy model (Wamsley & Zald, 1973; Zald, 1970) and the exchange or power-dependency model (Jacobs, 1974; Thompson, 1967).

The degree of dependence is measured by the extent to which an organization relies on another to attain its goals. The more dependent an agency is, the more it will communicate with others. Before an interorganization relationship develops, a focal organization must be aware of its system's needs, problems, or opportunities, and of the other agency's service and goals. Personal acquaintance of representatives of the organizations involved is also important.

Consensus among the organizations about solutions, services, and goals is the step that follows awareness. Similarity of domain with respect to goals, services, staff skills, and clients is a consideration in resource dependence research as is the number of agencies involved in the interactions.

Structure

Interorganizational relationships occur when resources are transmitted between two or more organizations. Money, physical materials, client referrals, technical staff services, and information are frequently exchanged resources. IOR exchange has been described at three levels: pairwise, organizational set, and organizational network. Most research has been at the pairwise or dyadic level (Aldrich, 1979; Hall, Clark, Giordano, Johnson, & Van Rockell, 1977; Klonglan, Warren, Winkelpleck, & Paulson, 1975; Litwak & Hylton, 1962). These studies focused on the direction and intensity of the transactions between two organizations. The organizational set consists of one focal organization and the other organizations in its environment with which it has direct links (Caplow, 1964; Evan, 1966). The concept of organizational set is based on Merton's role set (1957). Links in organizational sets are identified by the flow of resources between the focal organization and the organizations in its set and by boundary spanning activities.

An organizational set, which centers on a focal organization, differs from an action set that refers to an interacting group of organizations (Boissevain, 1974). The action set is analogous to a coalition in which a temporary alliance is formed to accomplish a purpose or project that a single organization can not handle alone. Action sets are frequently formed to lobby for legislation of mutual benefit to organizations. Once the objective is reached, the interactions between and among the action set decrease or cease.

The third structural level is the interorganizational network. It is the pattern of interrelationships of a cluster of organizations that functions as a social system to attain collective goals or to solve common problems (Jay, 1964). A network differs from the pairwise and organizational set levels in that it is constructed by identifying all the ties between and among all organizations in a population. An underlying assumption is that networks systematically inhibit or facilitate the activities of organizations at an aggregate level. Networks are usually represented in graph or matrix form.

In a graph, connecting arrows illustrate the structure of the influence exerted between and among organizations. Influence can be exerted directly or indirectly through other organizations. A matrix simply indicates the presence or absence of a relationship between organizations in a network.

Network analysis has been used to describe the spread of educational innovations (Clark, 1965), the diffusion of medical techniques and drugs (Becker, 1970; Coleman, Katz, & Menzel, 1957), the delivery of human service (Aldrich, 1978), and the management of multiorganizational emergency responses in search and rescue operations (Drabek, 1968; Drabek, Tamminga, Kilijanek, & Adams, 1981). Although networks are not corporate bodies that have set boundaries or that can take action, the concept of organizations being linked helps to clarify the conditions under which they will form coalitions or exchange resources.

In order to monitor and analyze the degree of dependence and the amount of exchange that occurs between and among organizations, researchers developed operational dimensions. Marrett (1971) developed and Aldrich (1979) adapted the structural dimensions of formalization, intensity, reciprocity, and standardization. These are summarized as follows.

Formalization or official recognition of transactions among organizations can occur by agreement or by structural change. Agreements can be mandated by legislatures or by bureaucratic directives. An example of this is the Block Grant legislation of 1981 that moved the administration of many health and human services from the federal to the state level. A more informal agreement would be represented by the referral that a community health nurse makes to a social service agency. Structural formalization refers to the extent to which a third party coordinates the relationships between organizations. Examples of this are the private recruitment organizations that locate nurse administrators for hospital employers or the coordinators who refer hospital patients to home care agencies.

Intensity is a measure of the investment that organizations have in their relationships with others. The amount of resources committed to a relation indicates its intensity. An example would be the number of referrals sent to a visiting nurse service by a medical center. Tangible resources such as money and goods are more easily quantified than are referrals. The frequency of interaction refers to the amount of contact organizations have with one another. Formalizing relations generally leads to more frequent interactions.

Reciprocity is the extent to which both parties benefit from the flow of resources or information. A dependence relation is marked by an asymmetrical exchange. As in the intensity dimension, the measurement of reciprocity is easier when the resource exchanged is money or goods. Definitional reciprocity refers to interactions whose terms are mutually agreed upon. Many relations are present because of regulations. For example, health departments are required to enforce health and safety regulations in eating establishments, nursing homes, and other facilities used by the public. In these cases, the dominating organization is a major determiner of whatever agreement is made with the dependent organization.

Standardization is a dimension related to traditional bureaucratic structure. Unit standardization is the extent to which the individual units in a transaction are similar. The more homogeneous the type of referrals to a home health agency, the more decentralized the decision making about the handling of the work (Perrow, 1967). Procedural standardization is defined as the degree of similarity in the transaction of procedures with another organization. People-processing organizations are less apt to have set procedures for transactions than are organizations that deal with nonhuman resources. Aldrich (1976a, 1976b) found that organizational size and complexity as well as intensity of interaction were correlated with standardized procedures.

Van de Ven and Ferry (1980) defined two other dimensions of IOR structure, complexity, and centralization. Complexity of IOR can be measured by the number of different resources exchanged and the number of subgroups involved in transactions. Centralization includes the locus of decision making and the information and resource flow. The locus of decision making is similar to Marrett's (1971) standardization dimension, described above.

In summary, the structural components include the levels of focus of IOR as well as the dimensions by which those relations can be measured operationally. In the next section, the processes or strategies that organizations employ in coping with their interdependence are described.

Process

A number of authors postulated that organizations attempt to reduce or absorb environmental uncertainty (Cyert & March, 1963; Hickson, Hinings, Lee, Schneck, & Pennings, 1971; Thompson, 1967). To cope with uncertainty, organizations are motivated to develop relationships with other organizations. Some prevalent coping behaviors used among interdependent organizations and the hoped-for outcomes of these interventions are discussed in this section.

A horizontal merger, in which two or more organizations come together under common control, is undertaken to maximize profits or avoid bankruptcy. This strategy is increasingly used in health care organizations, particularly hospitals. Such a merger may obliterate one organization's identity and/or may result in retention of the staff, facilities, and titles of the absorbed organization. Vertical integration, or merger, occurs when an organization acquires one of its suppliers or customers. An example would be a hospital that purchases its linen supply company.

Joint ventures are temporary alliances in which organizations pool part of their resources to carry out mutually beneficial tasks (Aldrich, Note 1). Joint ventures involve the relinquishment of less autonomy than horizontal mergers do. However, Paulson (1977) found that a maximum loss of autonomy occurred when coalitions (a form of joint venture) were formed to deliver health services.

Innovation refers to the introduction of new goods and services to enhance growth and improve market power (Pennings, 1981). Innovation is related to product differentiation. Hospitals that are horizontally dependent constantly seek to establish product differentiation by negotiating with physicians and other hospitals for domain consensus.

Regulations and licensure by the government protect existing organizations, such as hospitals, by restricting entry into the market. Certificates of need, building and zoning regulations, as well as third-party payor requirements inhibit the construction of health care facilities. Hospitals voluntarily apply for accreditation by the Joint Commission on the Accreditation of Hospitals (JCAH). This body can deny hospitals access to Medicare and Medicaid funds by withholding or withdrawing certification. Existing hospitals strive to comply with all regulations that might endanger their ability to survive.

Overlapping memberships occur when individuals connect two or more organizations, usually through memberships on boards of directors. Health care organizations frequently choose external directors to obtain financial, legal, or other information; to aid in the search for capital; and/or to enhance their political power. Directors may also be placed on hospital or health boards to enhance the public image of the organization that the director represents (Aldrich, 1979).

Organizational intelligence refers to gathering or distributing information, usually of a secret nature. Such information may assist organizations in forecasting what their competitors may be planning (LeBreton, 1969). Having advance information about a competitor's introduction of a new service may be of great value to a hospital organization. Boundary spanners frequently channel information about external development into their organizations. This information enables organizations to imitate successful innovations of competitors.

Flow of personnel through recruitment of executives and professionals from other organizations is a strategy that reduces developmental lags between organizations. Lieberson and O'Connor (1972), using time-series data, correlated leadership changes with performance measures such as sales and profit margins in large corporations. No similar studies were found for service organizations.

Antitrust suits are another coping strategy used to undo or prevent the growth of aggressive competitors. As more health care systems merge into larger and more powerful corporate structures, antitrust suits may become a more viable strategy for dealing with competition.

In an effort to make sense of IOR strategies, Paulson (1977) synthesized theory and research on health and welfare organizations. He developed a paradigm linking IOR solutions with the four functions of an organization (AGIL) defined by Parsons, Bales, and Shils (1953). These were mediated by autonomy and structure. For example, an administrator faced with the problem of acquiring patients in order to increase the organization's adaptation to the environment lost very little autonomy by bargaining with other agencies for referrals. The effect on the organizational structure of this combination, adaptation through bargaining, was increased centralization of decision making and decreased personnel loyalty within the organization.

Outcomes

As noted earlier, survival and adaptation to a changing environment are central problems of organizations. Haas and Drabek (1973) described the continuing struggle for autonomy, security, and prestige (ASP) as underlying the structure and process of organizational life. Although they were referring to the internal dynamics of an organization, the concepts of ASP are also desirable interorganizational outcomes. Security, which they equated with survival potential, depends on the possession of scarce resources. Prestige is related to an organization's rank relative to other organizations and to the respect and deference accorded by others. Prestige accorded an organization by its competitors is related directly to autonomy and survival.

In general, an organization's hierarchy of preferred IOR strategies is based on preserving autonomy. The most advantageous choice is a proprietary strategy in which organizational boundaries remain intact and ownership and control of resources are maintained. Proprietary strategies include aggressive actions such as hiring an executive from a competitor, price undercutting, gaining control over raw materials or distribution channels (vertical integration), product differentiation, or bribery of government officials (Aldrich, 1979).

Domain consensus is a desired outcome that contributes to the ASP of an organization. The strategy of product differentiation was described above as being related to developing domain consensus. Increased efficiency, effectiveness, coordination, market power, and growth, as well as decreased competition and rivalry are outcomes that have been alluded to above.

Pennings (1981) noted that organizations are motivated to develop coping strategies (processes) to coordinate their activities and to manage their interdependence (outcomes). He categorized the latter into forestalling, forecasting, and absorption. Forestalling prevents or controls other organizations' unpredictable behavior. Forestalling is accomplished through horizontal and vertical mergers, joint ventures, innovation, product differentiation, regulation, and overlapping. Forecasting, which predicts the behavior of other organizations, is accomplished by obtaining information about other organizations. Strategies include regulation, overlapping membership, organizational intelligence, and flows of personnel. Absorption, a reactive behavior, decreases the negative consequences of other organizations. This end is accomplished through horizontal mergers, regulation, overlapping membership, organizational intelligence, flows of personnel, licenses and imitations, and antitrust suits.

The discussion up to this point has pertained to the resource dependence perspective, which implies that organizations manipulate and select their environments. An alternative view is the population ecology framework, in which the unit of analysis is at the population or aggregate organization level (Aldrich, 1979). In this model, the environment is considered to have a role in shaping the design, mission, and strategy of organizations. Environments differentially select certain types of organizations for continuance, based on a fit between characteristics of the environment and organizational forms. For example, specialty hospitals for tuberculosis, crippled children, and maternity clients were superseded by large general hospitals. In the case of nursing education, hospital-based diploma schools were replaced by nursing programs in educational organizations or institutions.

Another interorganizational perspective is on the community. In community studies, investigators examined the relations that link a collection or set of organizations in a circumscribed geographic area. Emphasis was on the pattern or network of relations among organizations (Litwak & Hylton, 1962; Turk, 1971; Warren, 1967).

Methodological Concerns

A major deterrent to the development of IOR theory has been that the popular positivist research approach is not suitable. Experimental designs that stress the control of pertinent variables and assume independence from the external world are not useful in IOR that must take into account tremendous variety, continuous change and conflict, many confounding variables, and the tendency for organizations to adapt to their environments.

Another general problem is the choice of the unit of analysis and the appropriate aggregation of data. Lazarsfeld and Menzel (1969) developed a typology to distinguish between the properties of collectives and members. Collectives are comprised of members. The latter may be individuals, departments, organizations, or populations of organizations. The properties of collectives may be analytical, structural, or global, from which alternative inferences can be drawn. Analytical properties are obtained from measurements of members. An example would be that the average age of patients in a nursing home was 85 in 1981. This fact might be useful as a variable but does not give any information about the nursing home itself. The measurement of relationships among members forms the base for structural properties. Frequency of interaction between organizations in a network would be a structural property. Global properties are not based on member measures, but on collective characteristics such as economic assets or yearly budget. Global data cannot be used to describe members.

Member properties described by Lazarsfeld and Menzel (1969) were absolute, relational, comparative, and contextual. Absolute properties of members included information that is unrelated to the particular collective. An example would be the size of the organizations that compose a collective. Relational properties refer to such relationships among members as the intensity of interaction in a network of organizations. The pattern of intensity within the entire network would be a structural property of the network. Comparative properties of members are similar to absolute properties except that the value of the member is interpreted with reference to the distribution found in the entire collective. For example, the relationship between organizations A and B might be classified as the least complex relationship in an entire network. Contextual properties are collective characteristics that describe members. An example of a contextual variable would be that graduates of nonaccredited baccalaureate nursing schools frequently are denied entry into accredited master's programs in nursing.

The distinction between collective and member properties is useful in understanding when aggregation or disaggregation of data is appropriate. Aggregation is defined as the use of a combination of unit-characteristic (micro) responses to reflect or describe something about the immediately higher (macro) unit of analysis. The opposite is disaggregation, in which an aggregated mass is separated into its component particles (Roberts, Hulin, & Rousseau, 1978).

Shifts in levels of aggregation are most frequently criticized for their effects on statistical analyses that lead to errors in interpretation. "The fallacy of the wrong level" refers to the direct translation of properties or relations from one level to another, either by making inferences from groups downward to individuals, or by projection upward from members to the collective. "Ecological fallacy" (Galtung, 1967) is the term used for downward projection, that is, when characteristics of individuals are based on data from collectives. "The fallacy of aggregation" occurs when relationships on the member or individual level are assumed to apply on the collective level (Robinson, 1950). The research of Durkheim (1951/1895) on the relation of religion to suicide is an instance of a wrong level fallacy (Davis, 1961).

The development of measurement procedures for IOR research is not simple. The reality of organizations and their interactions must be inferred from relationships. What one desires to measure is not a concrete physical object. As Haas and Drabek (1973) noted, the treatment of data is probably more critical than the data base or the data source. In choosing measurement procedures, the investigator relies on the underlying theory and constructs that are to be explored.

Methodologies for IOR research are being developed. The confidence that can be placed on the early descriptive studies based on qualitative data is limited. Initially, researchers studied linkages between organizations simply by asking whether persons in two organizations knew one another. Over time, as the structural dimensions of IOR research were operationalized more fully, some researchers collected complex data and used sophisticated multivariate analysis techniques.

The relevance of the findings and techniques of social-psychological small-group research to interorganizational research is questionable. Interorganizational relations occur in open systems where boundaries cannot be controlled by researchers and where linkages may not be effective.

INTERORGANIZATIONAL RELATIONS RESEARCH PERTAINING TO NURSING

Although nursing care delivery systems interacted with other organizations and with their environment from their inception, a category entitled "interorganizational relations" does not appear in any list of nursing publications. Thus, a Medlars/Medline computer search of the literature yielded very few citations.

A search of the indexes of the journals of *Nursing Research* (1952 to 1981), *Western Journal of Nursing Research* (1979 to 1981), and *Research in Nursing and Health* (1978 to 1981) resulted in no articles with the term "interorganization" in the title. Searches of the Western Council for Higher Education in Nursing (WCHEN) *Proceedings of Communicating Nursing Research Conferences* (1968 to 1981) and of *Comprehensive Dissertation Indices A , Social Sciences* (1971 to 1981) brought to light a few interorganizational studies that related to nursing, health care delivery systems, or nursing education systems. Some relevant material was found in nonnursing journals and books.

For ease of presentation, the studies reviewed will be discussed under the headings of situational factors, structure, process, and outcome. There is considerable overlap, because a number of the investigators described linkages between and among the variables.

Situational Factors

The need for resources and for other agencies is a given. The need may be asymmetrical, may vary over time, and may not be recognized overtly, but it exists.

In several studies (Ahla, 1952; Dunbar, Munir, & Triplett, 1957), the necessity for nurses and social welfare workers to be aware of the other agency's unique contribution to the care of families was examined. These early investigations were atheoretical and descriptive. Galaskiewicz and Shatin (1981) investigated another aspect of awareness in a study of 181 human service and nonprofit organizations in four Chicago neighborhoods. Their hypothesis was accepted that when the environment is turbulent and uncertain, leaders of neighborhood organizations establish cooperative relationships based on their own personal neighborhood connections or status group affiliations.

Domain consensus and domain similarity were common themes for a number of nursing studies. Although Ahla (1952) used no conceptual framework, her conclusions were that the Visiting Nurse Association and the Family Service Agency served common clients, that each had a legitimate claim to the services it provided, and that nurses were health specialists and caseworkers were social specialists who dealt with family social disintegration. In a similar type of survey, Dunbar, Munir, and Triplett (1957) noted that social workers viewed nursing's domain as limited to physical problems, such as growth and development, and first aid. Offerman (1976) found that public agencies often were able to refrain from joint activities because of their ability to generate domain consensus about their functions.

A somewhat different study relating to consensus was done by Milio (1967). She found that a lack of value consensus between middle class health care providers and lower socioeconomic maternity clients led to prenatal care that was not in harmony with the beliefs and living patterns of those receiving care.

Several researchers examined degree of consensus in educator and employer perceptions of nursing education programs. Voight (1972) discovered that the educationally defined role of the technical nursing graduate was that of a provider of patient-centered care. The employers did not have a job description for a technical nurse, and they quickly programmed the associate degree graduate into a leadership role.

At the baccalaureate level, Canfield (1980) also noted incongruent perceptions on the part of nurse educators and employers. She found a statistically significant difference ($p < .05$) in their perceptions of the clinical competencies necessary for beginning critical care nurses in the clinical content taught in baccalaureate programs and in inservice programs offered by hospitals. Similarly, Knollmueller, White, and Yaksich (Note 2), in a survey of 526 public health nursing service agencies and 140 baccalaureate schools of nursing, found a lack of consensus in perceptions of student preparedness. A startling finding was that 38% of the agencies said that they would not hire new graduates of baccalaureate programs.

With two exceptions (Galaskiewicz & Shatin, 1981; Milio, 1967), the studies reviewed in this section were atheoretical. For the most part, they were descriptive surveys.

Structure

A case study of an organizational set consisting of a private hospital and its satellite charity hospitals was done by Milner (1980). Unlike Milio's finding that low income women were given care by middle class providers, Milner found that low income clients were referred to charity hospitals where the care was unequal. Milner's extrapolation from interpersonal interaction data to the organizational level is an example of the fallacy of aggregation, mentioned above as a methodological problem.

Schultz (1981) examined an organizational network in a comparative field study of primary care services in two rural Colorado communities. She described the effect on health care outcomes of the IOR among a network of health care providers, including public health nurses, physicians, dentists, pharmacists, and emergency medical technicians. Both the Milner (1980) and Schultz (1981) studies focused on the ways the recipient was influenced by the nature of the delivery system. Both implied that changes in the delivery system would alleviate problems of underserved populations. No studies were found that dealt with crucial higher level IOR, such as those between business and government agencies, between businesses, or between government agencies. It is at this level that conflicts among powerful actors determine such elementary health factors as safe water, food, air, drugs; type of care provider; and mechanisms for health care payment.

A few studies included references to the structural dimensions of IOR (Ahla, 1952; Chohan, 1978; Greene, 1976; Associated Hospital Services to New York, Note 3). All noted that formalization of interaction facilitated interorganizational coordination among community service agencies.

Greene (1976), in a natural field experiment, focused on informal client advocacy behavior in three hospitals serving hemodialysis and post-myocardial infarction patients. One agency formalized its patient advocacy by assigning a specific person to assist patients and family through the Medicare and Social Security maze. This formal boundary spanning role led to increased interagency referrals. A similar result was reported when the position of nurse coordinator was initiated in an economic feasibility study authorized by New York's Blue Cross-Blue Shield (Associated Hospital Services to New York, Note 3). Chohan (1978) hypothesized that complexity, centralization of decision making, and awareness of interdependence were associated with the decision to participate in a network. Interestingly, Chohan labeled awareness of interdependence as a psychological variable. This attribution of affective characteristics to an aggregate is of methodological concern.

Process

An excellent example of a horizontal merger is the unification model through which nursing service and nursing education have been brought under common control at the University of Rochester (Ford, 1980, 1981) and Rush-Presbyterian-St. Luke's Medical Center. The organizational framework of the Rush model is said to provide parity and shared power across nursing, medicine, administration, and the health sciences (Christman, Note 4). Little research has appeared in the literature concerning these horizontal mergers; studies of the effect of hospital mergers on nursing services have not been reported. Studies of vertical mergers and joint ventures or coalitions in nursing were not found. This was rather surprising, because these coping strategies frequently are used by nursing groups in the legislative arena. The continued expansion of the governmental relations efforts of the American Nurses' Association attests to the perceived necessity and value of forming coalitions around specific legislative issues.

Hanna-Boulos (1972) explored the relationship of certain organizational variables to the educational innovativeness of 18 publicly supported schools of nursing. Educational innovativeness correlated with such intraorganizational factors as degree of faculty participation in college affairs, influence over curriculum, faculty selection, and promotion. Innovativeness also correlated with the interorganizational factors of degree of interaction with the external environment and with number of external grants. This finding emphasizes the value of boundary spanning activities of faculty. Rushing (1971) examined the degree of success of governmental regulations designed to facilitate the coordination or to equalize the distribution of health care services. Using secondary data, median county family income, median education of county residents over age 25, and proportion of county men in professional organizations, Rushing found that the interdependence of these three variables led to the principle of cumulative advantage. That is, the stronger the community's economy and the better educated the population, the greater the community's chance to attract professional men, particularly physicians. This principle applied to regional medical programs, the Hill-Burton programs, Medicare, and Medicaid. Rushing's use of secondary data illuminated the lack of success of federal efforts to change health care delivery patterns. The vested interest groups that prevent or inhibit the use of such findings to change public policy were described by Alford (1975).

Collective bargaining between hospitals and unions was studied by Frank (1978). He tested the proposition that organizations establish interorganizational links to render a turbulent environment more stable and thereby enhance the organization's ability to control scarce resources. The turbulent environment resulted from the requirement that impassed contract disputes be submitted to arbitration for resolution. Formal and repeated exchange activity between hospital organizations enabled them to maintain control over wage levels, even with arbitration. Frank noted that arbitrators used prior wage decisions in other hospitals to establish wage disputes. The appropriateness of wage levels was influenced by gentlemen's agreements.

The most frequently reported IOR strategy used in nursing was the referral of patients (Ahla, 1952; Carn & Mole, 1949; Farrisey, 1954; Groscop, 1939–40; Joint Committee, 1947; Weisner & Murphy, 1944; New York State Association of Councils and Chests and the National Welfare Assembly, Note 5). The findings of all of these descriptive studies indicated the advantages of referrals to clients and agencies. Paulson (1977), in his synthesis of theory and research on IOR strategies used by health and welfare organizations, stated that an organization loses very little autonomy by bargaining with other agencies for referrals.

Outcome

Autonomy is a highly desired outcome of any interorganizational interaction. As just noted, many nursing studies have focused on the referral strategy that preserves agency autonomy.

Survival and prestige were major themes studied by Milner (1980). The survival of the higher status teaching hospital depended on controlling admission of patients needed for teaching and research purposes. At the same time, survival of the lower status satellites was contingent on referrals from the focal organization. Milner's interpretation of his findings was in harmony with those of Fennell (1980) and with the theoretical position of Alford (1975, p. 175) that dominant structural interests (professional monopolists and corporate rationalizers) create barriers to equality of health care.

Efficiency has been defined as the ability of an organization to minimize the cost of transforming resources into acceptable outcomes (Katz & Kahn, 1966). Efficiency, operationalized as low patient costs, was a factor that permitted agencies with low potential power to obtain United Way funding (Provan, Beyer, & Krytbosch, 1979). Similarly, the Associated Hospital Services to New York study (Note 3) indicated that increased use of visiting nurse services resulted in more efficient hospital usage.

Effectiveness refers to an organization's ability to acquire scarce resources from its environment. As with the concept of efficiency, referrals from hospital to home care were related to improved care and to more effective use of community resources (Carn & Mole, 1949; Joint Committee, 1947). In a more sophisticated action research project, Eller, Gordon, and Bradley (1958) found that early screening, diagnosis, and treatment could speed medical and economic recovery in families, particularly in cases assessed as having potential for rehabilitation.

Increased coordination of health services has been the reported outcome of IOR by a number of researchers (Jurkiewicz, 1980; Miller, 1979; Romo, 1971). Coordination has been defined as continuity of care (Farrisey, 1954), integration of services (Eller, Gordon, & Bradley, 1958; Weirich, 1978), cooperation (McCune, 1971), and participation (Chohan, 1978). This collective-level concept has been measured by asking informants (members) to name the organizations with which they had the most cooperative relationships in a given period. These exploratory descriptive analyses provide a base for more sophisticated research. One major deterrent to the use of the findings to change health care delivery systems is the absence of measurable cost benefit outcomes. Studies that included decreased competition and rivalry as outcome variables were not located.

Increased market power and growth have not been viewed as socially appropriate outcomes for health care agencies. However, they have been sought for reasons of survival, security, and prestige. Fennell's (1980) secondary analysis of Census data led to some interesting insights into the growth of hospitals. She found that as the proportion of elderly persons increased in a population, the range of services decreased and the number of nonprofit hospitals in a cluster increased. In addition, supplier diversity, operationalized as physician specialties, accounted for over 50 % of the variance in the range of services. She also found that to maintain prestige, hospitals duplicated services rather than expanding the range of services or providing higher quality or lower cost care. Her conclusion was that the actual consumers were not patients, but physicians and hospital administrators.

Fennell's use of Census data was a creative means of circumventing the fact that basic reliable descriptive data about health care institutions are scanty. (Fein, 1967; Freidson, 1972; Mechanic, 1972). The findings strongly supported Alford's (1975) position that professional monopoly (physicians) and corporate rationalization (administrators) are the major determinants of health care delivery in the United States.

The scarcity of nursing studies in the area of IOR was both a disappointment and a challenge. An attempt was made to include studies in this review with findings that seemed relevant to nursing, even if not specifically directed toward nursing organizations. The hope is that the material presented will stimulate nurse researchers to consider IOR research as a viable and tremendously vital field for study.

SUMMARY, RESEARCH DIRECTIONS

What started as a brief overview of interorganizational relations research (IOR) in the area of nursing and health care was expanded considerably when the definition rather than the term was used as the basis for selection of articles. Although no general theory of IOR research has gained wide acceptance, several frameworks have been developed that provide direction for research in the field. Perhaps a major value of this review is that it focuses attention on an area of study of high potential usefulness to nurse researchers and to nursing.

A recurring theme throughout the literature was that an awareness of the interdependency of organizations must precede the development of linkages that are mutually beneficial to the organizations and to the larger community/society system. Recommendations flow from a critical need to expand nursing's body of knowledge in the area of IOR. Studies are needed to describe the occurrence and relative effectiveness of strategies for coping with uncertainty that are used by nursing organizations. These strategies include mergers, joint ventures, innovations, referring, bargaining, contracting, sharing resources, and boundary spanning activities. Effectiveness could relate to the degree of autonomy, prestige, domain consensus, efficiency, or competition attained by an organization. The conceptual framework described in this chapter provides guidelines for developing numerous hypotheses related to nursing care delivery and nursing education systems.

Some suggestions for areas of further research follow:

1. The American Nurses' Association (ANA) and its linkages with other nursing organizations, e.g., the National League for Nursing, and nursing specialty organizations, as well as nonnursing groups

such as the American Hospital Association, the American Medical Association, and various national voluntary health organizations. (This is not a new idea. More than twenty years ago, the ANA Committee on Research and Studies [ANA, 1962] recommended research on the social context of nursing. Specific mention was made of the image and appraisal of ANA by members, nurse nonmembers, allied groups, and the public.)

2. The nursing education and nursing service organizations that are interdependent but may or may not be aware of the critical need to strengthen interorganizational relations.
3. Nursing service organizations of the same population type that increasingly will be expected to collaborate and cooperate rather than compete. Research delineating the effectiveness of strategies used by existing organizations could be used to initiate change.
4. Different populations of nursing organizations—acute care, long term care, community health nursing, and rehabilitation—need to define those linkages that lead to effective use of resources and to continuity of care.
5. Comparative studies of the economic value of different linkage strategies among nursing care delivery organizations and between nursing and other care-providing organizations seem critical to the future development of nursing.
6. The effectiveness of the unification models that have horizontally merged nursing education and practice need to be compared with other models for integrating nursing organizations.

An overall recommendation is that generalizations from IOR research be developed so that a scientific knowledge base in this area would be available for use by nurses in education, in practice settings, and, particularly, in administration.

REFERENCE NOTES

1. Aldrich, H. *Asian shopkeepers as a middleman minority: A study of small business in Wandsworth*. Paper presented at the annual meeting of the American Sociological Association, Chicago, 1977.
2. Knollmueller, R. M., White, C., & Yaksich, S. *Preparation for community health nursing in baccalaureate programs as viewed by nursing service admin-*

istrators and nursing educators. Report of special project. Service and Education Committee, Public Health Nursing Section. Washington D.C.: American Public Health Association, 1979.
3. Associated Hospital Services to New York. *Visiting nurse study: A study concerning the feasibility of providing nursing service to subscribers through visiting nurse agencies*. Interim report. New York: Author, 1955.
4. Christman, L. *The Rush model for nursing: Colleagues in patient care.* Announcement of conference/consultation, Chicago: Rush-Presbyterian-St. Luke's Medical Center, March 1, 1982.
5. New York State Association of Councils and Chests and the National Social Welfare Assembly. *The Utica study: Pilot study of local-national relationships among voluntary health and welfare agencies using Utica, New York, as the local base*. Utica, New York: Author, 1956

REFERENCES

Ahla, A. M. M. Referred by visiting nurse: A study of cooperation between the visiting nurse and the social case worker. *Nursing Research*, 1952, *1*, 37. (Summary)
Aldrich, H. Resource dependence and interorganizational relations between local employment service offices and social services sector organizations. *Administration and Society*, 1976, *1*, 419–454. (a)
Aldrich, H. An interorganizational dependency perspective on relations between the employment service and its organization set. In R. H. Kilman, R. Pondy, & D. P. Slevin (Eds.), *The management of organization designs* (Vol. 2). New York: Elsevier North-Holland, 1976. (b)
Aldrich, H. Centralization versus decentralization in the design of human service delivery systems: A response to Gouldner's lament. In R. Sarri & Y. Hasenfeld (Eds.), *Issues in service delivery in human service organizations*. New York: Columbia University Press, 1978.
Aldrich, H. *Organizations and environments*. Englewood Cliffs, N.J.: Prentice-Hall, 1979.
Alford, R. L. *Health care politics: Ideological and interest group barriers to reform*. Chicago: The Univeristy of Chicago Press, 1975.
American Nurses' Association Committee on Research and Studies. ANA blueprint for research in nursing. *American Journal of Nursing*, 1962, *62*, 69–71.
Becker, M. Sociometric location and innovativeness: Reformulation and extension of the diffusion model. *American Sociological Review*, 1970, *35*, 267–282.
Bendix, R. *Work and authority in industry*. New York: Wiley, 1956.
Boissevain, J. *Friends of friends: Networks, manipulation, and coalitions*. Oxford: Basil Blackwell, 1974.
Canfield, A. A comparison of the beginning level of clinical competencies for critical-care nurses as perceived by educators and employers. In *Communicating nursing research: Directions for the 1980s* (Vol. 13). Boulder, Colo.:

Western Interstate Commission for Higher Education, 1980. (Abstract)

Caplow, T. *Principles of organization.* New York: Harcourt, Brace, Jovanovich, 1964.

Carn, I., & Mole, E. W. Continuity of nursing care: An analysis of referral systems with recommendations. *Public Health Nursing,* 1949, *41,* 343–346.

Chohan, V. V. Organizational decision making and participation in an interorganizational service network (Doctoral dissertation, Portland State University, Oregon, 1978). *Dissertation Abstracts International,* 1978, *39,* 5173A. (University Microfilms No. 79–04, 284)

Clark, B. Interorganizational patterns in education. *Administrative Science Quarterly,* 1965, *10,* 224–237.

Coleman, J. S., Katz, E., & Menzel, H. The diffusion of innovations among physicians. *Sociometry,* 1957, *20,* 253–270.

Cyert, R. M., & March, J. G. *A behavioral theory of the firm.* Englewood Cliffs, N.J.: Prentice Hall, 1963.

Davis, J. A. *Great books and small groups.* New York: Free Press, 1961.

Dill, W. R. Environment as an influence on managerial autonomy. *Administrative Science Quarterly,* 1958, *2,* 409–443.

Drabek, T. *Disaster in Aisle 13.* Columbus, Ohio: College of Administrative Science, Ohio State University, 1968.

Drabek, T. E., Tamminga, H., Kilijanek, T. S., & Adams, C. *Managing multiorganizational emergency responses.* Boulder, Colo.: Institute of Behavioral Sciences, University of Colorado, 1981.

Dunbar, C., Munir, L. E., & Triplett, J. L. Social workers look at public health nursing. *Nursing Outlook,* 1957, *5,* 70–72.

Durkheim, E. *Suicide: A study in sociology.* (J. A. Spaulding & G. Simpson, trans.) New York: Free Press, 1951. (Originally published 1895.)

Eller, C. H., Gordon, H. H., & Bradley, B. Health and welfare issues in community planning for the problems of indigent disability. *American Journal of Public Health,* 1958, *48*(11, Part 2), 1–48.

Evan, W. The organization set: Toward a theory of interorganizational relations. In J. Thompson (Eds.), *Approaches to organizational design.* Pittsburgh: University of Pittsburgh Press, 1966.

Farrisey, R. M. Continuity of nursing care and referral systems. *American Journal of Public Health,* 1954, *44,* 449–454.

Fein, R. *The doctor shortage: An economic diagnosis.* Washington, D.C.: The Brookings Institution, 1967.

Fennell, M. L. The effects of environmental characteristics on the structure of hospital clusters. *Administrative Science Quarterly,* 1980, *25,* 485–510.

Ford, L. C. Unification of nursing practice, education and research. *International Nursing Review,* 1980, *27,* 178–183; 192.

Ford, L. C. On the scene: University of Rochester Medical Center—Unification model of nursing at the University of Rochester. *Nursing Administration Quarterly,* 1981, *6*(1), 1–9.

Frank, G. B. An interorganizational analysis of the industrial relations system of the Minnesota Hospital Industry (Doctoral dissertation, University of Illinois at Urbana-Champaign, 1978). *Dissertation Abstracts International,* 1978, *39,* 3168A. (University Microfilms No. 78–20, 936)

Freidson, E. The organization of medical practice. In H. E. Freeman, S. Levine, & L. G. Reeder, (Eds.), *Handbook of Medical Sociology* (2nd ed.). Englewood Cliffs, N.J.: Prentice-Hall, 1972.

Galaskiewicz, J., & Shatin, D. Leadership and networking among neighborhood human service organizations. *Administrative Science Quarterly*, 1981, *26*, 434–448.

Galtung, J. *Theory and methods of social research*. New York: Columbia University Press, 1967.

Greene, C. An analysis of health care teams: Services to patients with selected chronic disease processes. In M. V. Batey (Ed.), *Communicating nursing research* (Vol. 9). Boulder, Colo.: Western Interstate Commission for Higher Education, 1976.

Groscop, J. Committee to study relationships between official and non-offical public health nursing agencies. *American Public Health Association Yearbook*, 1939–1940, *10*, 118–122.

Guetzkow, H. Relations among organizations. In R. V. Bowers (Ed.), *Studies in behavior in organizations*. Athens, Ga.: University of Georgia Press, 1966.

Gulick, L., & Urwick, L. (Eds). *Papers on the science of administration*. New York: Institute of Public Administration, Columbia University, 1937.

Haas, J., & Drabek, T. *Complex organizations: A sociological perspective*. New York: Macmillan, 1973.

Hall, P., Clark, J., Giordano, P., Johnson, P., & Van Rockell, M. Patterns of interorganizational relationships. *Administrative Science Quarterly*, 1977, *22*, 457–474.

Hanna-Boulos, N. E. Organizational variables and innovativeness in collegiate nursing institutions: A comparative study (Doctoral dissertation, The University of Michigan, 1972). *Dissertation Abstracts International*, 1972, *33*, 5514A. (University Microfilms No. 73–06, 841)

Hickson, D., Hinings, C., Lee, C., Schneck, R., & Pennings, J. A strategic contingencies theory of interorganizational power. *Administrative Science Quarterly*, 1971, *16*, 216–219.

Jacobs, D. Dependency and vulnerability: An exchange approach to the control of organizations. *Administrative Science Quarterly*, 1974, *19*, 45–49.

Jay, E. The concepts of "field" and "network" in anthropological research. *Man*, 1964, *64*, 137–139.

Joint Committee on Integration of Social and Health Aspects of Nursing in the Basic Curriculum. Referral of patients for continuity of nursing care. *Public Health Nursing*, 1947, *39*, 568–573.

Jurkiewicz, V. C. An exploratory-descriptive study of interorganizational and case coordination programs for the multi-problem, frail, and minority elderly (Doctoral dissertation, University of California, Los Angeles, 1980). *Dissertation Abstracts International*, 1980, *41*, 94A. (University Microfilms No. 80–23, 326)

Katz, D., & Kahn, R. *The social psychology of organizations*. New York: Wiley, 1966.

Klonglan, G.,. Warren, R., Winkelpleck, J., & Paulson, S. Interorganizational measurement in the social sciences sector: Differences by hierarchical level. *Administrative Science Quarterly*, 1975, *20*, 434–452.

Lazarsfeld, P., & Menzel, H. On the relation between individual and collective properties. In A. Etzioni (Ed.), *A sociological reader on complex organizations*. New York: Holt, Rinehart & Winston, 1969.

LeBreton, P. *Administrative intelligence-information systems*. Boston: Houghton-Mifflin, 1969.

Levine, S., & White, P. Exchange as a conceptual framework for the study of interorganizational relationships. *Administrative Science Quarterly*, 1961, *5*, 583–601.

Lewin, K. *A dynamic theory of personality: Selected papers*. (D. K. Adams & Karl E. Zener, trans.). New York: McGraw-Hill, 1955. (Originally published 1935.)

Lieberson, S., & O'Connor, J. Leadership and organizational performance: A study of large corporations. *American Sociological Review*, 1972, *37*, 117–130.

Litwak, E., & Hylton, L. Interorganizational analysis: A hypothesis on coordination. *Administrative Science Quarterly*, 1962, *6*, 395–420.

March, J., & Simon, H. *Organizations*. New York: Wiley, 1958.

Marrett, C. On the specification of interorganizational dimensions. *Sociology and Social Research*, 1971, *56*, 83–99.

Mayo, E. *The social problems of an industrial civilization*. Boston: Graduate School of Business Administration, Harvard University, 1945.

McCune, D. An analysis of interorganizational cooperation in drug abuse programs (Doctoral dissertation, Stanford University, 1971). *Dissertation Abstracts International*, 1971, *32*, 4293A. (University Microfilms No. 72–06, 033)

Mechanic, D. Public expectations and health care: Essays in the changing organization of health service. New York: Wiley, 1972.

Merton, R. *Social theory and social structure*. Glencoe, Ill.: The Free Press, 1957.

Milio, N. Values, social class, and community health services. *Nursing Research*, 1967, *16*, 26–31.

Miller, P. An examination of interorganizational issues in coordination of human services (Doctoral dissertation, The Ohio State University, 1979). *Dissertation Abstracts International*, 1979, *40*, 4749A. (University Microfilms No. 80–01,.785)

Milner, M., Jr. *Unequal care: A case study of interorganizational relations in health care*. New York: Columbia University Press, 1980.

Offerman, B. Organizational characteristics, dependency, and joint programs: Mutual effects and correlates in interorganizational relations (Doctoral dissertation, Michigan State University, 1976). *Dissertation Abstracts International*, 1976, *37*, 3931A-3932A. (University Microfilms, No. 76–27, 139)

Parsons, T. *The structure of social action*. New York: McGraw-Hill, 1937.

Parsons, T. *Toward a general theory of action*. Cambridge, Mass.: Harvard University Press, 1951.

Parsons, T. *Structure and process in modern societies*. Glencoe, Ill.: Free Press, 1960.

Parsons, T., Bales, R., & Shils, E. *Working papers in the theory of action*. Glencoe, Ill.: Free Press, 1953.

Paulson, S. Interorganizational strategies for solving organizational problems: A synthesis of theory and research on health and welfare organizations. In E. H. Burack & A. R. Negandhi (Eds.), *Organizational design: Theoretical per-*

spectives and empirical funding. Kent, Ohio: Comparative Administration Research Institute, Kent State University, 1977.

Pennings, J. Strategically interdependent organizations. In P. C. Nystrom & W. C. Starbuck (Eds.), *Handbook of organizational design: Adapting organizations to environments* (Vol. 1). Oxford, England: Oxford University Press, 1981.

Perrow, C. A framework for comparative organizational analysis. *American Sociological Review,* 1967, *32,* 194–208.

Philips, A. A theory of interfirm organization. *Quarterly Journal of Economics,* 1960, *74,* 602–613.

Porter, L., Lawler, E., & Hackman, J. *Behavior in organizations.* New York: McGraw-Hill, 1975.

Provan, K., Beyer, J., & Krytbosch, C. Environmental link and power resource dependence relations between organizations. *Administrative Science Quarterly,* 1979, *26,* 200–225.

Roberts, K., Hulin, C., & Rousseau, D. *Developing an interdisciplinary science of organizations.* San Francisco: Jossey-Bass, 1978.

Robinson, W. Ecological correlations and the behavior of individuals. *American Sociological Review,* 1950, *15,* 351–357.

Roethlisberger, F., & Dickson, W. *Management and the worker.* Cambridge, Mass.: Harvard University Press, 1940.

Romo, J. An interorganizational study of psychiatrically disabled soldiers discharged from the U.S. Army and their subsequent relationship to the Veterans Administration (Doctoral dissertation, Brandeis University, Florence Heller Graduate School, 1971). *Dissertation Abstracts International,* 1971, *32,* 4117A. (University Microfilms, No. 72–01, 583)

Rushing, W. Public policy, community constraints, and the distribution of medical resources. *Social Problems,* 1971, *19,* 21–36.

Sahlins, M., & Service, E. *Evolution and culture.* Ann Arbor: University of Michigan Press, 1960.

Salancik, G., & Pfeffer, J. An examination of need-satisfaction models of job attitudes. *Administration Science Quarterly,* 1977, *22,* 427–456.

Scherer, F. *Industrial market structure and economic performance.* Chicago,: Rand McNally, 1970.

Schultz, P. Field study of rural primary care services: Their organization and effects (Doctoral dissertation, The University of Denver, 1981). *Dissertation Abstracts International,* 1981, *42,* 4949A. (University Microfilm No. 82–09, 946)

Selznick, P. *TVA and the grass roots.* Berkeley: University of California Press, 1949.

Selznick, P. *Leadership in administration.* New York: Harper and Row, 1957.

Stigler, G. *The organization of industry.* Homewood, Ill: Irwin, 1968.

Taylor, F. *The principles of scientific management.* New York: Harper, 1911.

Thompson, J. *Organizations in action.* New York: McGraw-Hill, 1967.

Turk, H. Interorganizational networks in urban society: Initial perspectives and comparative research. *American Sociological Review,* 1971, *35,* 1–19.

Van de Ven, A., & Ferry, D. *Measuring and assessing organizations.* New York: Wiley Interscience, 1980.

Voight, J. An exploratory study of the associate degree programs in nursing in selected community colleges in Michigan (Doctoral dissertation, The University of Michigan, 1972). *Dissertation Abstracts International*, 1972, *33*, 6041A-6042A. (University Microfilms No. 73–11, 288)

Wamsley, G., & Zald, M. *The political economy of public organizations*. Lexington, Mass.: Heath, 1973.

Warren, R. The interorganizational field as a focus for investigation. *Administrative Science Quarterly*, 1967, *12*, 306–419.

Weber, M. *The theory of social and economic organizations*. (A. H. Henderson & T. Parsons, Eds. and trans.). Glencoe, Ill.: Free Press, 1947. (Originally published 1924.)

Weirich, T. The politics of services integration: A study of change in interorganizational relations (Doctoral dissertation, Rutgers University, New Brunswick, N. J., 1978). *Dissertation Abstracts International*, 1978, *39*, 7010A. (University Microfilms No. 79–10, 452)

Weisner, D., & Murphy, M. Relationships of health agencies. *Public Health Nursing*, 1944, *36*, 39–43.

White, L. *The science of culture: A study of man and civilization*. New York: Farrar, Strauss, & Giroux, 1949.

Zald, M. Political economy: A framework for comparative analysis. In M. N. Zald (Ed.), *Power in organizations*. Nashville: Vanderbilt University Press, 1970.

Part III

Research on the Profession of Nursing

CHAPTER 8

Socialization and Roles in Nursing

MARY E. CONWAY

SCHOOL OF NURSING

MEDICAL COLLEGE OF GEORGIA

CONTENTS

There is no dearth of studies on the socialization of nurses. However, with the exception of a few researchers, notably Kramer (1968, 1970, 1972), no consistent conceptual view has been employed to guide such research. By far the largest amount of research on the socialization of nurses has centered on examining certain values and attitudes of graduating students in three types of nursing schools or measuring these same values and attitudes on a sample of nurses practicing in their first professional role. This latter fact prompts the question: Is the conceptualization of socialization, at least in the case of nurses, too limiting? Many scholars in the fields of sociology and psychology take the position that socialization is a continuing inter-active process between the person being socialized and the environment

183

(Brim, 1966; Clausen, 1968; Elkin & Handel, 1972; Goslin, 1969). Assessing a given population at any point in time to determine the degree of socialization representative of that population ignores the *process* of socialization. Whether it can be considered appropriate to measure attitudes and values toward the profession among about-to-be-graduated nurses and assume that these represent the "socialized" professional is even more debatable. What can such individuals know of the role they are about to assume other than that portrayed by teachers and a selected few practicing nurses whom they have observed during their clinical laboratory experiences? One assumption underlying such measurements is that the degree to which the neophyte subscribes to the values and norms of teachers can be considered a valid measure of socialization.

A variety of perspectives on the nature of socialization has guided recent research on the professional nurse role. A commonly held view of socialization for the world of work is that it is a specific kind of socialization, distinct from but not independent of socialization in general (Moore, 1969). Moore stated, "Socialization to the world of work may be for some a kind of conditioning, a reluctant preparation for harsh realities, and for others, a kind of commitment to a calling" (p. 862). Examples of these two conceptualizations of preprofessional socialization are represented by attitudinal items reported in the literature, particularly in research conducted by nurses themselves. Kramer (1970) exemplified the former perspective; Ondrack (1975) provided an example of the latter.

When either perspective guides a particular study, one must be skeptical in evaluating the conclusions drawn by the researcher. Does the choice of perspective bias the outcome? To what extent do the assumptions underlying the research question and/or the operational measures reflect researcher bias? For example, if the investigator assumes that professional practice and the bureaucracy are incompatible, are the test or interview items likely to focus heavily on the assumed areas of strain?

A further variant in the conceptualization of nurses' professional socialization is viewing socialization as an *outcome* of a prescribed program of formal training, as opposed to viewing training as the first stage of a career-long developmental process. Those holding this view (i.e., outcome) tend to use as indicators of successful outcome the extent to which the neophyte's values and perceptions of the nurse role are congruent with those of faculty or professionals already in practice. Research conducted by Crocker and Brodie (1974), Sharp and Anderson (1972), and Lynn (Note 1) are illustrative of an outcome view.

SOME PROBLEMS OF METHODOLOGY

A review of the research literature on socialization of nurses and their role development over the past ten years revealed that when selecting a study sample of practicing nurses, researchers have not always distinguished between nurses prepared at the technical level (i.e., in two- or three-year programs) and those prepared at the professional or baccalaureate level, at least when assessing such variables as commitment, role concept, role stress, role strain, and/or autonomy. In describing the demographic composition of a given sample, the researcher frequently reported the educational background of subjects, but less frequently used type of education as a control when examining scores on the dependent variable. An exception to this was found in a few studies in which the researcher stratified a sample of students with the intent of examining differences in values and attitudes, or role concept, that may relate to the type of educational program from which the sample was drawn. See Meleis and Dagenais (1981), for one example.

In organizing the research on socialization of nurses, one must cope with competing perspectives, methodological inadequacies, difficulties inherent in generalizing from limited or convenience samples, and inadequacies in conceptualization of the problem under study. There is the added problem that nursing research in general lacks a paradigm to guide it (Hardy, 1982).

An important question that has been asked repeatedly in research on socialization of nurses, one on which there has not been agreement, is: Is there a difference between the kind and level of competencies of graduates of professional and technical programs? Inadequate conceptualization of the problem can result in inadequate methodology. For example, asking faculty in each of the two types of programs to state what their expectations are for graduates of their programs does not answer whether the practice of these graduates differs.

One study that is noteworthy for the investigators' attempts to conceptualize the problem adequately and to measure actual differences in practice between graduates of associate and baccalaureate degree programs is that of Waters, Vivier, Chater, Urrea, and Wilson (1972). The investigators drew on characteristics in the literature that described both factual knowledge and intellectual processes required to practice nursing. In addition, the investigators observed two samples of nurses in actual practice in a hospital, each representing one type of educational background.

An evolutionary paradigm of the practice of nursing as reflected in role performance may come to guide later research. Evidence for this is seen in research aimed at describing role conceptualization of nurses for which instruments were constructed to measure traditional versus nontraditional views of the role. For example, in one study (Lynn, Note 1), subjects were asked to respond to statements that described various aspects of the nurse's role on a continuum of agreement, or alternatively, to discriminate between two statements, one which was a more traditional descriptor and one less traditional. Further, the large number of studies that were conducted on the so-called expanded role of the nurse seem to support the view that the role of the nurse evolved from some earlier set of role expectations to a newer configuration recognized by nurses and relevant others in a variety of practice settings.

An evolutionary paradigm would be consistent with the conceptualization of a system of roles, the view held by several persons (Conway, 1978; Katz & Kahn, 1966; Kuhn, 1974). Viewed as a systems phenomenon, an individual role is not independent but "related to the actions of others and to the state of other subsystems in the organization at any one point in time" (Conway, 1978, p. 112).

ORGANIZATION OF THIS REVIEW

Given the methodological issues identified above and the fact that the majority of studies conducted on socialization of nurses included multiple variables within a single study, this chapter has been organized as follows:

1. Socialization, further subdivided into those studies dealing with preprofessional and professional aspects of the socialization process, role performance, view of the profession, and expectations;
2. Role conception, including ideal role conception, sex-related role image, autonomy, and accountability; and
3. Sources of role stress, including role strain, role conflict, role clarity, and ambiguity.

Limitations of this review include the facts that the research reviewed spans a ten-year period, and women comprise the majority of subjects from which generalizations are drawn about socialization of nurses. A further limitation is the exclusion of research based on the so-called expanded role of the nurse. Although much of the research on the expanded role lacks a conceptual base, the role itself cannot be overlooked as one specialized aspect of socialization in nursing. However, because of space limitation and the absence of a conceptual framework generally, research on this role is not included in this chapter.

Three major data bases were generated as a guide to the selection of pertinent literature; the bases were drawn from ERIC, Medline, and *Psychological Abstracts*. In addition, seventeen professional journals and monographs were examined. This process of identification of pertinent research produced a total of 102 titles that were deemed "possibly relevant." Out of these, sixty-six of the most relevant were read and critiqued, and these formed the basis for this chapter.

A CONTINGENCY THEORY OF SOCIALIZATION

One piece of research (Feldman, 1976) is unique in attempting to understand which variables actually influence the process of socialization. Drawing on the literature, Feldman constructed a model with four stages of socialization: Anticipatory Socialization, Accommodation, Role Management, and Outcomes (p. 434). Variables assumed to operate at each stage were identified; for example, initiation to the task and role definition were presumed to occur in Stage II, Accommodation.

Feldman further identified four process and eight outcome variables that he measured following interviews with 118 employees in a medium-sized hospital. The initial sample on which final scales of the contingency model were constructed included engineers, radiology technologists, accounting clerks, nursing technicians, and registered nurses. He found that job satisfaction was relatively high for both engineers and nurses. His explanation was that both types of professionals had jobs suited to their skills and abilities. A difference between these two groups was that nurses had a great deal of difficulty in defining their jobs and as a consequence experienced role conflict.

Feldman's model offers a challenge for other researchers. While Feldman's idea of process and outcome seems an appropriate way to conceptualize socialization, his assumption that there is a *causal* order of process variables is less tenable. Feldman himself admitted that while he asserted a causal order, the research did not test the assumptions of the model. The potential of the model for use in further studies on the process of socialization into the world of work for nurses and others lies in its clearly delineated stages and the possibility for determining the extent to which certain variables operate at each stage.

PREPROFESSIONAL SOCIALIZATION

The research literature on preprofessional socialization revolves around three persistent questions: What image or expectations do students have of the profession they are about to enter? To what extent do students' attitudes and role concepts mirror those of the faculty who teach them? Are there differences in self concept and/or role concept among students in the three major types of educational programs?

Research on practicing professional nurses has reflected emphasis on the following questions: What is the professional concept of nurses? To what extent is there tension between the professional orientation of the nurse and the bureaucracy in which the majority are employed? What factors influence commitment to a (nursing) job? Are there any differences in the practice of nurses related to type of nursing educational program, and, if so, what are they?

In the introduction to this chapter, the author raised the question whether socialization should be viewed as a continuous or discontinuous process and speculated whether one view or the other would make any real difference in an analysis of the research on socialization, for the world of work. The author's bias is that socialization in general is properly viewed as a continuous process. While the author makes an assumption of continuity, for purposes of manageability, the research conducted primarily on students is reviewed in one section and that conducted on nurses in practice in another.

Socialization of Students: Process and Outcomes

A substantial amount of research on student nurses' role concepts has centered on determining the extent to which students' concepts match those of faculty and, in a few instances, the extent to which they are consistent with the role concepts of practicing nurses (Crocker & Brodie, 1974;

Ondrack, 1975). The inferences made from these studies were that the closer students' attitudes and values match those of their teachers or nurses in practice, the more complete or successful socialization has been. A difficulty in drawing generalizations from such research was the fact that some samples of students were drawn from any one of the different types of educational programs, while others contained students from a variety of programs: diploma (DI), associate degree (AD), and baccalaureate (BS). A further limit upon generalizability was that nearly all of the samples were local or regional and of relatively small size. The use of a variety of tools to test professional role concept, some of which had no reported reliability and validity, further limited generalization.

Findings from research done prior to 1977 indicated that there were few real differences in the role concept, attitudes, and expectations regarding future work roles among seniors in all types of programs. Later research revealed findings of major differences. Meleis and Farrell (1974) studied 188 students drawn from each of three types of programs in San Francisco and attempted to identify biographical and attitudinal differences among senior students. Ten subscales were used, including measures related to (a) value placed on research, (b) leadership qualities, (c) autonomy, and (d) self-esteem. The instruments used to measure these variables included a research scale adapted from Rosinski (1963), the Leadership Opinion Questionnaire of Fleishman (Note 2), the Autonomy Scale from the Omnibus Personality Inventory (Heist & Yonge, 1968), and the Self-Esteem Test (Barksdale, Note 3).

Based on scores that yielded differences on two variables, Meleis and Farrell concluded that there were more similarities than differences among students from these programs. The differences were that AD and BS students scored higher on autonomy than did DI students, and DI students placed a higher value on research than students from the other two programs.

Tetreault (1976) studied BS junior and senior students (N = 157) in one school of nursing to assess whether teacher beliefs were adopted by students. She defined "message" factors and "teacher" factors as variables in the interactive process between teachers and students. Two hypotheses tested were: (a) when teacher professional attitude is high, students are likely to score high on a professional attitude measure, and (b) when teacher consideration of students is high, students will have higher professional attitude scores. The questionnaire that was administered included three instruments: the Instructor-Leader Behavior Questionnaire (Dawson, 1972), Hogan's Professionalism Test (1972), and an investigator-constructed semantic differential instrument to measure beliefs on "what is" and "what should" the profession be. Instrument validity and reliability were not reported. The "message" hypothesis was supported, but "only students who were highly challenged by teachers" showed a tendency to accept the message (p. 51). Students who rated teacher consideration high had significantly higher scores on professional attitude. A surprising finding was that there was no difference between junior and senior students in their views of the profession as both an active and positive force.

Ondrack (1975) compared attitude changes in students in three hospital-based diploma schools. He made the assumption that "socialization in professional schools is a function of attitude and value consistency among significant others during the socialization process" (p. 97). He conceptualized a process model of socialization in which inputs were entering students, the process consisted of attitudinal cues provided by significant others (teachers and nurses in clinical settings where students had experience), and outputs were more or less positive socialization. The Nurse Attitude Questionnaire (NAQ), consisting of seven attitude scales, was administered to a sample of students, teachers, head nurses, and practicing staff nurses in three hospitals.

In phase one of the study, each school and hospital was assessed for degree of internal consistency. In school A, teachers and staff nurses differed on only two of seven subscales of the NAQ and in school C, faculty and staff nurses differed on six out of the seven subscales. Thus school A was judged to have high internal consistency; school C was judged to have very low consistency. School B fell between schools A and C on total scores. Students were chosen nonrandomly. Teacher, head nurse, and staff nurse participation was described as voluntary. Students in school A (high consistency) scored close to their teachers at graduation on five of seven attitude scales of the NAQ, while students in school C (low consistency) differed significantly from their teachers on these same scales. Differences between students and teachers in each of the two schools were established by pretest at time of entrance. No such consistent trend toward or away from teacher attitudes was found in school B (moderate consistency). No reliability or validity for the scales was reported.

In another study, Crocker and Brodie (1974) measured the degree of congruence between students' and faculties' scores on a multivariate instrument representing diverse views (expectations) of the profession. Using a convenience sample of 488 students in a midwestern BS program, they constructed an instrument composed of 112 behaviors common to practicing nurses (Nurses' Professional Orientation Scale). Items were obtained by interviews with hospital-employed nurses. These 112 items were rated for importance by 94 instructors; the final scale consisted of 60 items. Response categories measured the extent to which opinions of students shifted toward those of faculty during their academic preparation. Students' views shifted markedly toward those of faculty, with a significant spread between the scores of freshmen and seniors. Scores of seniors were numerically close to those of faculty. An important methodological step in this research, one missing in a number of other studies purporting to assess degree of socialization upon graduation, was the validation of nursing behaviors based on practicing nurses themselves. However, a problem of internal validity was that faculty whose only clinical practice was limited to the supervision of students during the latter's clinical laboratory experience may not model accurately for students the professional role of the practicing nurse.

In another study, Sharp and Anderson (1972) sampled 117 nursing students in one BS program in order to ascertain whether "successful and unsuccessful freshmen nursing students differed in their descriptions of the ideal nurse" (p. 340). The Gough and Heilbrun (Note 4) Adjective Check List (ACL) of 300 personal attitude items was used. Freshmen, sophomores, juniors, seniors (N = 117) and faculty (N = 14) completed the instrument. For analysis freshmen were divided into successful and unsuccessful subgroups; the unsuccessful subsequently transferred from nursing or were dropped from the program. Scores on the ACL did not discriminate between successful and unsuccessful candidates. Little difference was found between the scores of freshmen, upperclassmen, and faculty. In general, all students scored higher than faculty on deference ($p < .01$), and faculty scored higher than sophomores and freshmen on autonomy ($p < .01$). The investigators concluded that "students of nursing in order to be successful, need to adopt a professional role model similar to that held by their faculty" (p. 342). Whether this conclusion was supported by the research is open to question. Since there were very small differences in scores on the ACL between faculty and students at all ranks, a more plausible conclusion is that those students who already held attitudes similar to nursing faculty chose the nursing major. As other research has shown, students are likely to move closer to faculty in their personal conceptions of the ideal nurse as they advance in their academic program.

Some Differences: Reports of Recent Studies on Students

In studies conducted in the 1960s on personality characteristics of nurses, investigators reported nursing students to be more submissive, self-abasing, and to have lower needs for dominance and achievement than other college women (Bailey & Claus, 1969; Gortner, 1968; Psathas & Plapp, 1968). Some contradictory findings were reported independently by Stein (1969) and Gunter (1969) which in retrospect appear to herald a change in previously described characteristics of nursing students. Stein (1969), using the Edwards Personal Preference Scale (1957), found that students had higher needs for heterosexual relationships and autonomy than had been found among nursing students in earlier research. Gunter (1969), using Shostrom's (Note 5) Personal Orientation Inventory (POI), found that sophomore students were more mature than a normative sample of female freshmen college students on inner directedness, existentiality, aggression, self-acceptance, and capacity for intimacy.

Studies completed between 1976 to 1982 confirmed that the earlier role concepts attributed to students in BS programs did not describe students of this latter period. In one sample of 163 students divided among AD, BS, and DI seniors about to graduate, Meleis and Dagenais (1981) reported that when measured by a standardized instrument, nurses scored much like other college women. Two instruments were used in this research: the authors' Nurse's Self-Description Form (NSDF) and the male/female identity scale from the Omnibus Personality Inventory (Heist & Yonge, 1968). Validity and reliability were established for both instruments. The major findings reported by Meleis and Dagenais were that: (a) nursing students with high feminine sex identity expressed feelings of aggressiveness (unlike students in earlier studies); (b) self-descriptors were related significantly to program affiliation and not to sex role identity; and (c) AD and BS nurses scored significantly higher on the professional subscale of the NSDF than did DI students ($p < .01$). While one must be cautious about generalization when subjects were drawn from schools in only one city and the sample size was small, some confidence is justified that these findings are representative of a change in the traditional professional role concept held by nursing students. Further, the Meleis and Dagenais data on measures of self knowledge and professionalism clearly differentiated between students in the diploma school and those in the other two schools.

Findings reported in the literature on students' professional orientation are not uniformly consistent. Stromberg (1976), using a measure of sex role identity, reported that when students' sex role identity was more masculine, the students' image of nursing was "more in harmony with the image advanced by the profession" (p. 363). Tetreault (1976), in a sample of nursing students in the upper division, investigated the amount of relative agreement between students and their teachers on items descriptive of the profession. She reported high similarity between the students' concept of the profession and that of their teachers, particularly when the variable of teacher consideration was high. Lynn (Note 1) studied differences in professional orientation among students (N = 276) from selected AD and BS programs in the southern part of the United States. She found the AD nurses were more traditional in their view of nursing; but there were no differences between the two groups' scores on the Nurses' Professional Orientation Scale (Crocker & Brodie, 1974). Given these reported inconsistencies, before sound generalizations can be made both about students' professional orientation and differences in orientation between those in technical and professional nursing programs, it will be necessary to employ standard measuring instruments for which construct validity has been established.

SOCIALIZATION AND ITS CORRELATES AMONG NURSES IN PRACTICE

In the time period 1972 to 1982, six recurrent problems appeared in the research literature on socialization of nurses in practice. These were: (a) role conception, (b) autonomy, (c) role conflict, (d) role strain, (e) ambiguity, and (f) differentiation between the practice of professional and technical nurses, the BS and AD/DI. The theoretical basis for the majority of studies that were examined had been drawn from previously published work on the individual in the organization. Explicit and/or implicit assumptions were that individuals generally were more satisfied with their work and more committed to the organization, if they perceived that they had control over their work. A further assumption was that job satisfaction was related to both role clarity and moderate or low role strain (Snoek, 1966). The variable of medical dominance must be considered when examining the practice of nurses and the amount of discretion they have in their roles. Medical dominance as a limitation upon the practice of health professionals in general has been well documented by Freidson (1970).

Role Conception

Benner and Kramer (1972), in a sample of 162 baccalaureate nurse graduates employed in special care units, hypothesized that these nurses would have both higher professional role conceptions and higher bureaucratic role conceptions than other nurses. A third hypothesis was that special care unit (SCU) nurses would demonstrate higher integrative behaviors. In part, the theoretical rationale was that SCUs require more technically focused than expressive actions, and thus more conflict between the professional versus bureaucratic orientation could be expected. It was theorized that to reduce role deprivation, subjects would employ so-called integrative behaviors.

The empirical relevance of the findings of this study, had they been in the direction predicted, was that such nurses would have less role deprivation and therefore be more likely to remain longer in such positions. Corwin's Role Conception Scale (1961) and Kramer's Role Behavior Scale (1970) were used to assess role concept and extent of integrative behaviors. While no validity or reliability coefficients were reported for Kramer's scale, it is purported to assess behaviors that allow for adherence to both bureaucratic and professional role ideologies. The first two hypotheses were not supported by the findings, but the third was (Benner & Kramer, 1972). The possibility of these subjects' sensitization to testing must be considered, because this sample of nurses had served as subjects in earlier research by Kramer (1970).

Davis and Underwood (1976) interviewed a small sample ($N = 44$) of psychiatric nurses practicing in community mental health agencies. Using an investigator-designed interview schedule to assess respondents' views of their roles, the investigators found that these nurses had a limited view of the overall role and functions of the community mental health nurse. Their views appeared to be based more on "what they did" as opposed to the possibilities for intervention in the larger field of mental health practice. The subjects included nurses who possessed the BS degree and those who had no degree. Those with more education saw themselves as having more input into decision making and policies than did the others.

Kellberg (1972) studied a small sample of nurses, the majority of whom were diploma graduates, to determine whether nurses employed in coronary care units (CCU) differed from other nurses. From a random sample of 60 nurses among 15 hospitals, Kellberg selected 15 working in CCUs and 15 working in general units as controls. Subjects were queried via telephone interview regarding their learning objectives, satisfaction with their work, and the amount of communication they had with other professionals. Kellberg found that both groups of nurses expressed a high degree of satisfaction with their work. She failed to find support for the working hypothesis that coronary care nurses experienced an additional socialization process not shared by other nurses.

Bevis (1973) reported on a study in which role conception was the independent variable and participation in continued learning the dependent variable. Using Corwin's (1961) scale, Bevis tested 106 female, BS nurses employed in 23 midwestern hospitals to determine their role orientations. Subjects completed a Job Activity Survey (JAS) consisting of 110 items, 47 of which were "educational" in nature. No reliability or validity was established for the instrument. Each subject was rated as high or low on bureaucratic, professional, and service orientation. The dependent variable was total time a subject spent in educational activities in the first year of employment. Three hypotheses were tested: (a) nurses scoring higher than others on professional role concept would have significantly greater participation in continuing education activities; (b) there would be equal participation in continuing learning activities for both high and low service-orientation subjects; and (c) extent of participation in continuing learning would be related more to role concept than to personal characteristics. The first hypothesis was supported, but hypotheses two and three were not. Generalizability of these findings is not possible, because the sample was nonrandom, and neither validity nor reliability was assessed for the JAS. There is also a question about whether inducements or rewards in any of the subjects' job settings were used to encourage (or discourage) continued learning. For example, might a reward such as a merit increase motivate participation in continued learning regardless of the role orientation of the nurse?

A methodological study by Minehan (1977) is noteworthy for its attempt to determine the conceptual validity of the Corwin (1961) scale, the most widely used scale prior to 1979 to categorize role orientations of nurses. Minehan posited that Corwin's conceptual definitions did not describe adequately then current nursing practice. The expressed purpose of this study was "to develop a contemporary instrument which could be utilized with nurses employed in an urban teaching hospital" (p. 375). The results were intended to be used as a guide for the hospital-based educational presentations for nurses. Minehan's findings were inconclusive. Twenty-seven new items were included in her scale, each built on an underlying item in the Corwin scale, but only six correlated significantly with the comparable Corwin item. Following varimax rotation to determine item clusters, the emergent clusters were *not* those that had been designed to measure the designated role concept. Her methodology pointed up the questionable practice of attempting to assess construct validity of a new scale by the "known group" method—the method employed by some in scale development. Minehan did not claim validity for her own scale, but use of it by other investigators should help to determine the validity and reliability.

Autonomy

Autonomy, the amount of discretionary control the individual has over the performance of actions in the course of practice, has been a frequent topic for research. Autonomy is a condition of practice claimed or aspired to by the "completely" socialized professional. Alexander, Weisman, and Chase (1982) examined selected organizational determinants of perceived autonomy and the characteristics of the work setting that influenced nurses' perceptions of their jobs. The structural features selected for study included: (a) unit workload, (b) rank of the staff nurse, and (c) requirement for shift work. In a sample of 798 staff nurses in one university hospital, with BS, AD, and DI nurses represented, Alexander, Weisman, and Chase found that possession of the BS degree related significantly to perceived autonomy ($r = .13, p < .05$). Subjects who had received positive evaluations from head nurses scored higher in autonomy than others ($r = .34, p < .05$). Internal locus of control as measured by Rotter's (1966) I-E Scale was associated positively with autonomy.

In a three-factor analytic study of nurse autonomy, patients' rights, and rejection of traditional role limitations, Pankratz and Pankratz (1974) found that nurse leaders and those possessing the BS and master's degree scored higher than others on all three scales. Subjects in this study ($N = 702$) were representative of a community hospital, a university hospital, and a specialty (psychiatric) hospital. When controlling for setting, a direct linear correlation for all three factors was found with (a) advanced education, (b) leadership, (c) academic setting, and (d) nontraditional social climate (the specialty hospital).

Haller (Note 6), exploring the relationship between individual control over practice and innovation in the hospital setting, surveyed 720 hospital-employed nurses in 1977 and 684 in 1978. Thirty hospitals in Michigan were represented. The investigator's theoretical basis for examining the relationship was that "there is a known relationship between autonomy and expertise, and a logical necessity for an innovation process to intervene between the development of new knowledge and its expert use in practice" (p. 269). A stratified probability sample was employed to select hospitals from which subjects were drawn. Both construct validity of the items and discriminant validity by alpha test were reported for the instrument. Items were selected from the Crane, Pelz and Horsley (Note 7) Conduct and

Utilization of Research in Nursing Questionnaire. With perceived control over practice the independent variable, Haller reported that the greater the perceived control, the greater the perceived responsibility of the individual to innovate ($r = .34, p < .01$). In those hospitals where nursing had been categorized by the investigator as more influential, the administrators expressed a greater responsibility for innovation than their peers in the hospitals where nursing had been categorized as less influential. Haller's operational measure of autonomy merits scrutiny. Autonomy was measured by a four-factor index: (a) feeling responsible, (b) satisfaction with one's work, (c) participation in decisions, and (d) taking initiative. The index was the weighted sum of these four measures. As a matter of both conceptual and empirical clarity, it is difficult to conceive of "satisfaction" as a measure of autonomy. While satisfaction with one's work may be related to autonomy, it would appear to be related as a dependent variable rather than a contributor to autonomy.

Conway, Kirk, and Oliver (Note 8) investigated autonomy within the context of intentional change in professionals' practice. The theoretical basis of the study was diffusion theory. The investigators examined under what conditions adoption of innovation became the responsibility of the individual practitioner. Subjects were drawn by systematic random sample of nurses and social workers listed in the national membership rolls of the respective professional organizations. On the assumption that the amount of control one perceives one has over one's practice might be related to taking initiative to change that practice, two Likert-type response items intended to elicit self-perceived autonomy were included in the questionnaire. There were differences in scores on autonomy, but no significant within-group differences for changers and nonchangers. A limitation of this study was the possibility that the sample was not representative because not all practitioners are members of their professional association.

Weisman, Alexander, and Chase (1981), seeking to discover factors related to job turnover among hospital staff nurses, made the assumption that a number of factors, both personal and endogenous, were related to job turnover. They constructed a path analysis model assuming noncausal covariation between personal and job-related attributes. Autonomy was treated as one of several endogenous variables. The survey instrument consisted of the Job Descriptive Index (Smith, Kendall, & Hulin, 1969) to measure job satisfaction and four items from the Quality of Employment Survey (Quinn & Shepard, Note 9) to measure autonomy. Both short job tenure and low job satisfaction correlated significantly with turnover. Autonomy emerged as the strongest predictor of job satisfaction.

Hinshaw's (1975/1976) investigation of decision making by professional nurses warrants consideration here even though autonomy per se was not the variable measured. Hinshaw studied the task discretion exercised by nurses, and to the extent that task discretion is an integral component of professional autonomy, the findings from this study provided mixed information. Task discretion was defined as the amount of control one has over one's duties. Hinshaw constructed two theoretical models within which she hypothesized decision selection by nurses could be predicted. There were (a) the organizational model, focusing on routineness or complexity of tasks and (b) the professional model, relating decision selections to prior socialization of the practitioner. In a sample of 88 registered nurses, employing a magnitude estimation technique (Stevens, 1960), Hinshaw tested a number of hypotheses. Four are reported here. Within the frame work of the organizational model, the hypothesis that both task frequency and task discretion influence search decisions negatively was supported. A second hypothesis, that task complexity influences discretion negatively, was not supported. A third hypothesis, tested within the professional model, that task complexity would exert a strong positive effect on search intensity, was supported. A fourth hypothesis within this model was that discretion would have a positive effect on search intensity; findings were in a direction opposite to that predicted. In terms of the inferences that can be drawn about task discretion (autonomy) and its relationship to nurses' decisions on the basis of these findings, the most that can be said is that the amount of discretion exercised is a function of the interaction of both organizational and professional factors operating in a given setting. The mixed findings in this study may be related in part to an imperfect conceptualization of how professional and organizational values interact to influence the behaviors of individuals.

Role Conflict and Role Strain

The recurrently reported shortage of hospital nurses over the decade has spawned a small body of research aimed at discovering the salient subjective and structural factors that may contribute to dissatisfaction with the role of hospital nurse. Such terms as "burnout" and "reality shock" recur in the literature written by nurses themselves. It is not clear whether these catchwords describe real phenomena or whether they are expressions of frustration over circumstances in the work setting beyond the individual's control. Friction between the professional in attempts to maintain some degree of autonomy over work and the demands of the organization is a phenomenon long recognized as indigenous to all bureaucratic settings, one not experienced by nurses alone. A review of the research literature reveals the factors studied most frequently to include role stress, role strain, and role conflict. Role ambiguity is considered a component of role strain. Presumably, the more successful preprofessional socialization is, the better prepared the practitioner will be to deal with role stress, role strain, and role conflict.

Role stress was defined as a general term encompassing a variety of sources of role strain, including role ambiguity, role conflict, role incongruity, and role overload (Hardy, 1978). The subtleties of the distinction between role stress and role strain are of less concern in this review than the phenomena themselves; thus both terms will appear here, with usage depending upon the individual investigator's definition of the term.

Davis (1974) investigated whether intrarole conflict contributed to job satisfaction among a small sample of psychiatric nurses. Intrarole conflict was defined as the discrepancy between the activities and decisions the nurse expects to participate in and the expectations of that participation held by physicians and patients. Methodology had two parts: physicians and patients in a psychiatric unit of a hospital were asked how much involvement nurses should have in a certain aspect of care such as physical care, psychotherapy, and ward milieu; nurses alone responded to the Brayfield and Rothe (1951) Job Satisfaction Scale. Davis reported a significant difference between physicians' and nurses' expectations and between patients' and nurses' expectations of appropriate functions for nurses. High intrarole conflict existed in the sample, but contrary to expectations, high intrarole conflict was not associated with lower job satisfaction.

Feldman (1976), testing his own model of socialization, sampled 118 hospital employees, of which 22 were nurses. He found little role conflict in his subjects but found that nurses did not fit the general pattern of other employees. That is, nurses scored higher on a three-question measure of conflicting demands, and nurses were less successful in resolving conflicting demands. His explanation was that "nurses have the severest role conflicts to handle at work managing the conflicting demands of medical and administrative duties, and at home managing unusual scheduling problems and the effects of patients' problems on them" (p. 446). By contrast, engineers and radiology technicians had few such conflicts.

In a study designed to identify organizational and nonorganizational determinants of nurse turnover in two large university-affiliated hospitals, Weisman, Alexander, and Chase (1981) identified at least six major variables, role strain among them, that were associated with job satisfaction and turnover. Variables classified as components of role strain were: inappropriate physician delegation of tasks, workload, and professional time adequacy. Each of these variables was associated significantly with job satisfaction and intent to leave the job. The theoretical framework for the study was a causal model in which employee turnover was viewed as the "joint product of individual characteristics and the attributes of their jobs and work organizations" (p. 432). Autonomy and job satisfaction were viewed as intervening variables, with turnover and intent to leave being the two dependent variables. The operational measure of job satisfaction was the Job Descriptive Index (Smith, Kendall, & Hulin, 1969), and intent to leave was the number of times a nurse reported that she was "seriously looking" for a job. By path analysis coefficients and regression equations, similar outcomes were found in each setting. On the basis of R^2 values, the results were reported to be in the predicted direction.

Brief, VanSell, Aldag, and Melone (1979) examined the relationship between anticipatory socialization and role stress in a random sample of 157 registered nurses in Iowa. There were approximately equal numbers of BS, AD, and DI graduates. The authors' assumption was that each of the three types of programs "comprise distinct socialization processes that lead to different role conceptualizations" (p. 162). If this were the case, the investigators reasoned, there would be disparities between the anticipated role and reality of role demands on neophytes. A mailed questionnaire comprised of four scales was sent to all respondents. The four scales included: the Calkin (Note 10) Activity Inventory; the Rizzo, House and Lintzman (1970) Role Conflict/Ambiguity Scale; the Smith, Kendall, and Hulin (1969) Job Descriptive Index; and the Brayfield and Rothe (1951) Job Satisfaction Index. It was hypothesized that role stress for the general duty hospital nurse would vary with type of basic educational program. Results of a one-way analysis of variance, controlling for type of program, supported the hypothesis ($p \leq .05$). While role conflict and ambiguity were highest for graduates of BS programs, there were no within-group differences with respect to task activities. Since the measures of role stress in this study were general rather than specific, the basis for the findings of higher role stress among BS nurses is unknown. The investigators attributed it to underutilization of nurses' education. Whether or not underutilization was the "cause" of role stress, the investigators' conclusion that role expectations which are not congruent with demands of the setting are a source of role stress seems justified.

Conway (1977), who employed a convenience sample of 79 nurses in one governmental hospital and 64 controls in another in investigating the extent to which nurses were willing to assume accountability, found that role strain was lower for those subjects who scored higher than others on a measure of work-related autonomy. It was hypothesized that self-actualization or personal autonomy would be associated with less role strain, but no hypothesis had been formulated relative to work-related autonomy and role strain. Role strain was measured by the Snoek (1966) Job Related Tension Index (JRT). The JRT has reported reliability and validity. Construct validity was established for the author's index of autonomy.

Lyons (1971) examined the relationship between need for role clarity and role strain, assuming that greater anxiety and job tension would result from ambiguous roles. Lyons measured associations between role clarity and job satisfaction and between role tension and both propensity to leave the job and rate of voluntary withdrawal from the job. A sample of 165 nurses in a 400-bed hospital were differentiated on a measure of self-assessed need for role clarity. Both a role clarity and a need-for-clarity index were constructed by the investigator to achieve this differentiation. Role clarity (independent variable) was associated inversely with role strain, regardless of subjects' scores on need-for-clarity. Regardless of the magnitude of subjects' need-for-clarity, the higher the subjects' self-reported role clarity, the lower their role strain ($p < .01$). Reliability and validity for the indexes were not reported.

In a study in which commitment to the organization was the dependent variable, Hrebiniak and Alutto (1972) examined the effects of the variables: (a) intention to seek advanced formal education, (b) role strain, (c) role ambiguity, and (d) authoritarianism. Measurement instruments included the California F Scale (Adorno, 1950); Organizational Tension and Role Ambiguity Scale (Kahn, Wolfe, Quinn, Snoek, & Rosenthal, 1964); the Hrebiniak and Alutto (1972) six-item Interpersonal Trust Scale; and an author-constructed Commitment Index consisting of 12 items to elicit attitudes toward the employing organization. The sample consisted of elementary and secondary school teachers ($N = 318$) and hospital-employed registered nurses (N = 395). No between-group difference in commitment scores was found. Role strain was correlated inversely with commitment ($p < .01$). In an analysis of variance, role strain and length of service in the organization were the two variables that accounted for the greatest amount of variance in commitment.

The foregoing studies established role strain as an important factor in the employment setting for nurses. Role strain is closely linked to job satisfaction, even though intervening variables may exist. The practical implications of these findings are, or should be, of concern to nurses and their employers. In future research on role strain and job satisfaction, there is a need to identify specific sources of role strain. The data are insufficient to support the claims that role expectations generated during the process of education are a cause of role strain and/or conflict in the employment setting, at least not more for nurses than for other professionals employed in formal organizations.

Competencies and Type of Educational Preparation

The research reported in this section is presented in the order of the historical appearance of the studies. Noteworthy for its theoretical framework, comprehensiveness, and appropriate methodology was the study conducted by Waters, et al. (1972). The purpose of the study was to "attempt to document some differences in practice between graduates of baccalaureate and associate degree programs" (p. 124). The theoretical framework included selected characteristics from the literature that described both factual knowledge and the intellectual processes required for the practice of nursing. The investigators examined three aspects of practice: (a) the nature of problems practitioners solve and characteristics of the decision-making process, (b) scope of practice, and (c) attitudes of the practitioner toward practice. Methodology consisted of interviews with twelve directors of nursing and twenty-two head nurses in twelve hospitals in one large urban area to determine if they perceived any differences in the practice of the two types of nurses. All head nurses identified differences, and all but two directors of nursing distinguished differences between the two types of nurses. The differences were in the nurses' identification of problems, initiative, and their approach to solving problems. BS nurses acted independently in their approaches to patients' problems.

A further methodological step was the interviewing of two samples of nurses: 25 AD graduates and 24 BS graduates. Each of these nurses was observed for a period of time (a minimum of 30 minutes) and then interviewed about the first clinical incident requiring a decision that was observed by the researcher. Interviews were taped and coded by two expert judges. The interviewer in each instance explored with the subject the three aspects of practice identified above. Major differences reported by the investigators were that the BS nurses were self-directed, willing to take risks, dependent on self in most decisions, considered patients' social and psychological needs, and both saw and acted on the obligation to educate others. The AD nurses, by contrast, identified mainly physical or physiological problems of patients, and the actions they took had predictable outcomes. A limitation of this study was that there were no precise operational definitions of technical and professional nursing to guide the data collection. Major strengths of this study were its adequate conceptualization of the problem and the appropriateness of its design, particularly the attempt to assess the reliability of interview responses by observing nurses in practice.

Chamings and Teevan (1979) investigated the "expected competencies" of BS and AD nurses, gathering their data by means of interviews with directors of both types of programs, 63 BS and 56 AD. Using 80 items from a taxonomy of competencies (N = 234) developed prior to their investigation by the Southern Regional Education Board (Haase, Note 11), they asked: (a) Are there differences in overall level of competencies? (b) Should differences be expected in the kinds of competencies? The 80-item competency list represented three major clusters of competencies: human, conceptual, and functional. The investigators reported finding significant differences on 82 % of the items. Specifically, directors of BS programs had higher expectations for their graduates on both the conceptual and human subscales than did directors of AD programs. Both BS and AD directors expressed no differences in expectations for either group on the functional subscale. The investigators concluded that there were no differences in expectations regarding kinds of competencies. An inherent difficulty and possible threat to validity in constructing "competence" items for nurses lies in the fact that directors of associate degree programs who, among others, judge such items generally themselves have advanced degrees in nursing and/or education. Thus their expectations regarding kinds of competencies appropriate to AD graduates may reflect their own professional socialization rather than what might be more appropriate for a technically prepared practitioner. In addition, the tendency of employing agencies to use the graduates of each type of program interchangeably reinforces this blurring of distinction between technical and professional preparation.

Boss (Note 12) reported using factor analysis to arrive at a single criterion of job competence for nurses. Her method included a national sampling of 1,038 nurse faculty from 85 nurse-preparing programs. All three types of educational programs were equally represented. Respondents were asked to judge the importance of the items contained in two rating scales: Clinical Nurse Rating Scale (Reekie, 1970/1971) and the Nurses' Professional Orientation Rating Scale (Crocker & Brodie, 1974). The respondent pool in each type of educational program was split in half; one group was used in the factor analysis to determine the items' underlying dimensions, and the other group served as the cross validation sample to test the homogeneity of subscales. In an orthogonal varimax rotation, five principal factors emerged which were categorized within a cognitive-leadership and an interpersonal dimension. While factor analysis yielded several clearcut dimensions of expected competencies in the nurses' practice, no single criterion adequately measured all dimensions of competent practice. Boss reported no significant differences in the dimensions by type of program faculty.

An obvious limitation of this study was that two performance rating scales were employed, and there was no assurance that these scales contained all of the competencies required for successful nursing practice. In addition, the judgments were those of educators, not of practicing professionals. A question meriting consideration in the area of evaluating competence is whether the utilization of scales measuring entry level into the profession is appropriate. That is, does entry level competence constitute the entire dimension of professional practice in nursing? In terms of one question raised at the outset of this review, are socialization, and competence, to be considered complete at the time of the neophyte's entry into practice? Common sense would indicate that such is not the case. This study pointed up, as have others, the need to identify competencies based upon the practice of successful practitioners and to construct rating scales based on these known variables. This is a much needed next step in further research on the socialization of nurses.

SUMMARY

Suggested directions for future research have been identified in each section of this review; hence no attempt is made to repeat them here. What is clear is that research to date has not demonstrated conclusively that there is a difference in either the expected or actual competencies of practicing nurses as related to type of educational program. Primary sources of role stress for professional nurses that have been documented repeatedly include ambiguity, lack of autonomy, and limitations imposed on the development of the nurses' professional role by the competing demands of the work setting and other professionals, notably physicians. Still unknown are the critical variables that contribute to "complete" socialization and their relative contribution to the socialization of those nurses who are judged successful in the performance of their roles.

REFERENCE NOTES

1. Lynn, M. R. *The professional socialization of nursing students: A comparison based on type of educational program.* Paper presented at the annual meeting of the American Educational Research Association, Los Angeles, Calif., April 1981. (ERIC Document No. ED 201268)
2. Fleishman, E. A. *Manual for leadership opinion questionnaire.* Chicago: Science Research Associates, 1969.
3. Barksdale, L. S. *Building self esteem.* Unpublished manual, 1972. (Available from Barksdale Foundation for Furtherance of Human Understanding, Los Angeles, Calif.)
4. Gough, H. G., & Heilbrun, A. B. *The adjective check list manual.* Palo Alto, Calif.: Consulting Psychologists Press, 1965.
5. Shostrom, E. L. *EITS manual for the personal orientation inventory.* San Diego, Calif.: Educational and Industrial Testing Service, 1966.
6. Haller, K. Control over practice: Its relationship to innovation in hospital nursing departments. Baltimore: *Proceedings Fifth Biennial Eastern Conference on Nursing Research,* 1982.
7. Crane, J., Pelz, D., & Horsley, J. A. *Conduct and utilization of research in nursing.* Research instrument, 1977. (Available from University of Michigan, School of Nursing, 1335 Catherine Street, Ann Arbor, MI 48109.)
8. Conway, M., Kirk, S., & Oliver, N. Do professionals change their practice? Baltimore: *Proceedings Fifth Biennial Eastern Conference on Nursing Research,* 1982.
9. Quinn, R., & Shepard, L. J. *The 1972–1973 quality of employment survey.* Ann Arbor: Institute of Social Research, University of Michigan, 1974.
10. Calkin, J., Wallace, R., Chewning, B., & Gustafson, D. *Project to improve the utilization of nurses in ambulatory care settings* (Technical Report). Madison: University of Wisconsin, Health Services Engineering, 1975.
11. Haase, P. T. *A proposed system for nursing: Theoretical framework,* Part 2. Unpublished report. Atlanta, Ga.: Southern Regional Education Board, 1976.
12. Boss, B., *Perceived dimensions of nursing practice: A factor analytic study using more educators.* Paper presented at the Annual Meeting of American Educational Research Association, Los Angeles, Calif., April 1981. (ERIC Document No. ED 201264)

REFERENCES

Adorno, T. *The authoritarian personality.* New York: Harper, 1950.
Alexander, C., Weisman, C., & Chase, G. Determinants of staff nurses' perceptions of autonomy within different clinical contexts. *Nursing Research,* 1982, *31,* 48–52.
Bailey, J. T., & Claus, K. E. Comparative analysis of the personality structure of nursing students. *Nursing Research,* 1969, *18,* 320–326.

Benner, P., & Kramer, M. Role conceptions and integrative role behavior of nurses in special care and regular hospital nursing units. *Nursing Research*, 1972, *21*, 20–29.

Bevis, M. E. Role conception and the continuing learning activities of the neophyte collegiate nurse. *Nursing Research*, 1973, *22*, 207–216.

Brayfield, A. H., & Rothe, H. F. An index of job satisfaction. *Journal of Applied Psychology*, 1951, *35*, 307–311.

Brief, A., VanSell, M., Aldag, R., & Melone, N. Anticipatory socialization and role stress among registered nurses. *Journal of Health and Social Behavior*, 1979, *20*, 161–164.

Brim, O. G. Socialization through the life cycle. In O. G. Brim, Jr., & S. Wheeler (Eds.), *Socialization after childhood: Two essays*. New York: Wiley, 1966.

Chamings, P. A., & Teevan, J. Comparison of expected competencies of baccalaureate and associate degree graduates in nursing. *Image*, 1979, *11*, 16–19.

Clausen, J. A. (Ed.). *Socialization and society*. Boston: Little, Brown, 1968.

Conway, M. Accountability and its acceptance by professional nurses. In M. V. Batey (Ed.), *Communicating nursing research*, (Vol. 8). Boulder, Colo.: Western Interstate Commission for Higher Education, 1977.

Conway, M. Organization, professional autonomy and roles. In M. Hardy & M. Conway (Eds.), *Role theory: Perspectives for health professionals*. New York: Appleton-Century-Crofts, 1978.

Corwin, R. Role conception and career aspirations: A study of identity in nursing. *Sociological Quarterly*, 1961, *2*, 69–86.

Crocker, L. M., & Brodie, B. J. Development of a scale to assess student nurses' views of the professional nursing role. *Journal of Applied Psychology*, 1974, *59*, 233–235.

Davis, A., & Underwood, P. Role, function and decision making in community mental health. *Nursing Research*, 1976, *25*, 256–258.

Davis, M. K. Intrarole conflict and job satisfaction on psychiatric units. *Nursing Research*, 1974, *23*, 482–488.

Dawson, J. E. Effect of instructor-leader behavior on student performance. *Journal of Applied Psychology*, 1972, *56*, 369–376.

Edwards, A. L. *Techniques of attitude scale construction*. New York: Appleton-Century-Crofts, 1957.

Elkin, F., & Handel, G. *The child and society: The process of socialization*, (2nd ed.). New York: Random House, 1972.

Feldman, C. A contingency theory of socialization. *Administrative Science Quarterly*, 1976, *21*, 433–452.

Freidson, E. *Professional dominance*. New York: Atherton, 1970.

Gortner, S. R. Nursing majors in twelve western universities: A comparison of registered nurse students and basic senior students. *Nursing Research*, 1968, *17*, 121–129.

Goslin, D. A. (Ed.). *Handbook of socialization theory and research*. Chicago: Rand McNally, 1969.

Gunter, L. M. The developing nursing student: Part 3. A study of self appraisals and concerns reported during the sophomore year. *Nursing Research*, 1969, *18*, 237–243.

Hardy, M. Role stress and role strain. In M. Hardy & M. Conway (Eds.), *Role theory: Perspectives for health professionals.* New York: Appleton-Century-Crofts, 1978.

Hardy, M. Metaparadigms and theory development. In N. Chaska (Ed.), *The nursing profession: A time to speak.* New York: McGraw-Hill, 1983.

Heist, P., & Yonge, G. *Omnibus personality inventory—form F.* New York: Psychological Corporation, 1968.

Hinshaw, A. S. Professional decisions: A technological perspective. (Doctoral dissertation, University of Arizona, 1975). *Dissertation Abstracts International,* 1976, *36,* 7635A. (University Microfilms No. 76-11, 334)

Hogan, C. A. *Registered nurses' completion of a bachelor of science degree in nursing: Its effect on their attitude toward the nursing profession.* Unpublished master's thesis, St. Louis University, 1972.

Hrebiniak, L. G., & Alutto, J. Personal and role related factors in the development of organizational commitment. *Administrative Science Quarterly,* 1972, *17,* 555–573.

Kahn, R. L., Wolfe, D., Quinn, R., Snoek, D., & Rosenthal, R., *Organizational stress: Studies in role conflict and ambiguity.* New York: Wiley, 1964.

Katz, D., & Kahn, R. *The social psychology of organizations.* New York: Wiley, 1966.

Kellberg, E. R. Coronary care nurse profile. *Nursing Research,* 1972, *21,* 30–37.

Kramer, M. Nurse role deprivation: A symptom of needed change. *Social Science and Medicine,* 1968, *2,* 461–474.

Kramer, M. Role conceptions of baccalaureate nurses and success in hospital nursing. *Nursing Research,* 1970, *19,* 428–439.

Kramer, M., McDonnell, C., & Reed, J. L. Self-actualization and role adaptation of baccalaureate degree nurses. *Nursing Research,* 1972, *21,* 111–123.

Kuhn, A. *The logic of social systems.* San Francisco: Jossey-Bass, 1974.

Lyons, T. F. Role clarity, need for clarity, satisfaction, tension, and withdrawal. *Organizational Behavior and Human Performance,* 1971, *6,* 99–110.

Meleis, A., & Dagenais, F. Sex-role identity and perception of professional self in graduates of three nursing programs. *Nursing Research,* 1981, *30,* 162–167.

Meleis, A., & Farrell, K. Operation concern: A study of nursing students in three nursing programs. *Nursing Research,* 1974, *23,* 461–468.

Minehan, P. L. Nurse role conception. *Nursing Research,* 1977, *26,* 374–379.

Moore, W. E. Occupational socialization. In D. A. Goslin (Ed.), *Handbook of socialization theory and research.* Chicago: Rand McNally, 1969.

Ondrack, D. A. Socialization in professional schools: A comparative study. *Administrative Science Quarterly,* 1975, *20,* 97–103.

Pankratz, L., & Pankratz, D. Nursing autonomy and patients' rights. *Journal of Health and Social Behavior,* 1974, *15,* 211–216.

Psathas, G., & Plapp, J. Assessing the effects of a nursing program: A problem in design. *Nursing Research,* 1968, *17,* 336–342.

Reekie, E. Personality factors and biographical characteristics associated with criterion behaviors of success in professional nursing (Doctoral dissertation, University of Washington, 1970). *Dissertation Abstracts International,* 1971, *31,* 5212A. (University Microfilms No. 71-8534)

Rizzo, J., House, R., & Lintzman, S. Role conflict and ambiguity in complex organizations. *Administrative Science Quarterly,* 1970, *15,* 150–163.

Rosinski, E. F. Professional, ethical and intellectual attitudes of medical students. *Journal of Medical Education*, 1963, *38*, 1016–1022.

Rotter, J. B. Generalized expectancies for internal versus external control of reinforcement. *Psychological Monographs*, 1966, *80*, (1, Whole No. 609).

Sharp, W. H., & Anderson, J. C. Changes in nursing students' descriptions of the personality traits of the ideal nurse. *Measurement and Evaluation of Guidance*, 1972, *5*, 339–344.

Smith, P. C., Kendall, L., & Hulin, C. L. *The measurement of satisfaction in work and retirement*. Chicago: Rand McNally, 1969.

Snoek, D. Role strain in diversified role sets. *American Journal of Sociology*, 1966, *71*, 363–372.

Stein, R. F. The student nurse: A study of needs, roles, and conflict. *Nursing Research*, 1969, *18*, 308–315.

Stevens, S. S. The psychophysics of sensory functions. *American Scientist*, 1960, *48*, 226–273.

Stromberg, M. F. Relationship of sex role identity to occupational image of female nursing students. *Nursing Research*, 1976, *25*, 363–369.

Tetreault, A. Selected factors associated with professional attitudes of baccalaureate nursing students. *Nursing Research*, 1976, *25*, 49–53.

Waters, V., Vivier, M. L., Chater, S., Urrea, J. H., & Wilson, H. S. Technical and professional nursing: An exploratory study. *Nursing Research*, 1972, *21*, 124–131.

Weisman, C. S., Alexander, C., & Chase, G. Determinants of hospital staff nurse turnover. *Medical Care*, 1981, *19*, 431–443.

PART IV

Other Research

CHAPTER 9

Philosophic Inquiry

ROSEMARY ELLIS
FRANCES PAYNE BOLTON SCHOOL OF NURSING
CASE WESTERN RESERVE UNIVERSITY

CONTENTS

Nursing research predominantly has developed through the use of research and theory construction processes in empirical science. Much of the knowledge needed for professional nursing practice is of the nature of empirical science. There are other ways of knowing, however, other realms of meaning that are also important in nursing. Philosophy is one of these realms. It is another important way of knowing.

The knowledge base for nursing practice includes empirical science, but it also must include clarification of values, ethics, and study of the nature of knowledge or ways of knowing essential to professional nursing practice. A few nurses have engaged in philosophic inquiry in the quest for nursing knowledge. The *potential* contribution of philosophy to nursing knowledge development has been recognized. As yet it has not been realized.

Silva (1977) wrote of the need to examine the role of philosophy in deriving nursing knowledge. She identified three implications for nursing research pertaining to the inherent interrelatedness of science, theory, and philosophy. The following statements quoted from Silva present her thesis.

1. Ultimately all nursing theory and research is derived from or leads to philosophy.

211

2. Philosophical introspection and intuition are legitimate methods of scientific inquiry.
3. Nursing knowledge arrived at by the scientific method too often sacrifices meaningfulness for rigor. (pp. 61–62)

Silva addressed the relationships among philosophy, theory, and science. She also exposed the limitations for nursing of overemphasis on scientific method and rigor before a philosophical stance is established and significant nursing questions are identified and considered. Current activity in model building and grand theories of nursing practice are searchings for meanings and philosophic stance.

Beckstrand (1978) identified logic and ethics, both of which are branches of philosophy, as components of nursing knowledge and later (1980) noted that "many aspects of philosophy are entailed in the knowledge used in nursing" (p. 78). Carper (1975/1976), in her philosophic inquiry, identified ethics as one of four fundamental patterns of knowing that are found in nursing literature. Her own inquiry demonstrated the contribution, not limited to ethics, that philosophical investigators can make in nursing. A report of a part of the Carper investigation has been published (Carper, 1978).

The need for philosophic inquiry arises not simply from the need for logic and ethics or from the need for study of the nature of knowledge, but also from philosophic questions called forth by the fundamental nature of nursing. Such questions as the following must always be considered by nurses. What does it mean to be human? What is the meaning of dignity? What does it mean to be compassionate, humane, and caring? What is nursing? Such questions cannot be answered from the data or facts of science. They cannot be studied by impersonal, objective experimentation. The questions are sweeping, broad in scope, and value-laden; they defy final answers. They are questions professional nurses cannot ignore. Philosophic inquiry is the avenue by which nurses can address such questions.

Philosophic inquiry is inquiry to extract or clarify meanings from existing knowledge. It is used to make manifest and to clarify values; to identify ethics; and to study the nature of knowledge. Scientific research is a search for new formulations. It arises from the need for new knowledge and inadequacies in knowledge. It is done for some purpose that is tied to the perspective and beliefs of the investigator. Philosophic inquiry is used to expose, clarify, and articulate the perspectives, beliefs, conceptualizations, and methods that characterize a field. Through philosophic inquiry, scholars attempt to make known the good or desirable and the effective means to such ends. Philosophic inquiry makes explicit perspectives, methods, and the norms for the acceptable.

However one chooses to answer the philosophical question of what is nursing, it is apparent that the goals of nursing are the health and welfare of humans. These goals, as Curtin (1979) pointed out, are not scientific; they are moral. They are a seeking of good. They call for philosophic inquiry to clarify means and ends.

In attempting to articulate goals and modes for attaining goals, nurses have philosophized about nursing. Philosophies of nursing have been written for over a century. Many present-day theories or models are more philosophies of nursing or philosophic perspectives than theories or models from science. Most of these theories or models have not been developed or communicated in the method of philosophy. The theories or models have been attempts to articulate the essence of nursing, to identify desired goals, the good. Their authors showed their beliefs about the nature of human beings, human potential, and nursing. The models are individual statements of the oughts of nursing; they are projections of the desirable. They convey beliefs and stances toward some purpose. They are products of wisdom, experience, intuition, introspection, and values. They are not products of scientific or formal philosophic inquiry. They are sometimes called philosophies of nursing in the common usage "philosophy" but not in the usage of "philosophy" as a discipline.

Philosophy as a discipline is concerned with eternal problems such as the relation between mind and body or the nature of knowledge (Rorty, 1979). Philosophers endeavor to see reality as a whole. They analyze the nature and findings of different branches of knowledge; they examine the assumptions on which they rest and the problems to which they give rise. Philosophers seek to establish a coherent view of the whole domain of experience (Kneller, 1978).

Phenix (1964), in his system for the logical classification of realms of meaning, identified philosophy as a synoptic field, comprehensive in scope.

It is concerned with every kind of human experience and not with any one domain . . . All dimensions of all kinds of experiences come within its purview . . . The distinctive function of philosophy is the interpretation of meaning . . . *The meanings expressed in philosophy are meanings of meanings. . . .*

The method of philosophy is essentially that of dialectic, a process of conceptual examination, examination by raising questions, proposing answers, and developing implications of those answers in continuing cycles . . . In philosophic inquiry the question is more important than the answer, for the answer, if accepted as beyond question, stops inquiry. [Phenix, P. H. *Realms of Meaning*. New York: McGraw-Hill, 1964, p. 253, 254. Used with permission.]

Philosophy seeks explication of meanings, not measurement of concepts. It provides logical, semantic, and conceptual analyses, not formulations or reformulations to organize facts or to generate new theories. It is argumentative, directed at examination of presuppositions and implications, and at the determination of what logical relations do or do not obtain (Flew, 1979).

Carper (1975/1976), in her philosophic study of ten years (1964 to 1974) of nursing textbooks and journals, noted the shift in nursing language from observational to conceptual. Conceptualizations, conceptual analyses of various sorts, concern for ethics and values, and for essential meanings are now common in nursing literature. More formal philosophic inquiry is clearly appropriate and essential in nursing. The purpose of this chapter is to review the philosophic research that has been done by nurses from the first study by Newton in 1949 to February 1982.

The usually identified branches of philosophy are epistemology, that branch that investigates the origin, nature, methods, and limits of human knowledge; metaphysics; logic; and ethics. These branches did not prove useful for organizing a review of nursing research. No studies of nursing or by nurses were found to be in the branches of metaphysics or logic. Only the Carper (1975/1976) study could be considered as epistemology, and only two studies, those of Sternberg (1979) and Norberg, Norberg, and Bexell (1980) dealt with ethics. Philosophic studies done by nurses were studies of nursing using the methods of philosophy. They are useful for nursing. They are not classifiable by any single branch of philosophy. They also cannot be classified by any formal taxonomy for nursing research that exists.

In the absence of an established system for organization of the comprehensive field covered by philosophic inquiries in nursing, organization, for purposes of this review, was created by four general areas in which nurses were found to have made formal inquiry as philosophers. The review will be presented under general headings for the four areas; (a) ethics; (b) philosophy of nursing education; (c) concepts, values, and processes; and (d) methodology. These areas are not necessarily mutually exclusive. Some studies touched upon more than one area. The areas do serve to group studies and present a general picture of nursing research that stems from philosophy.

ETHICS

General societal concerns for ethics and the implications of developments in science and technology have resulted in growing attention to ethics in general, to bioethics or biomedical ethics, to ethical issues in human rights and human experimentation, and to professional ethics.

Investigations pertinent to ethics are beginning to appear in the nursing literature. Applegate (1981), Davis (1981), Ketefian, (1981a, 1981b), and Murphy, (1976/1977) are empirical studies of nurses or students in nursing. These studies were not philosophical inquiries and are not reviewed here. The Mooney (1980) study of ethical components in four nursing theories also was not a formal philosophic inquiry. Only two studies in this area were found that qualify as formal philosophic inquiry, those of Sternberg (1979) and Norberg, Norberg, and Bexell (1980).

Sternberg (1979) undertook a search for a conceptual framework as a philosophic base for nursing ethics. Sternberg defined ethics as the philosophy concerned with morality, its problems and judgments. Ethics is concerned with how one uses morality in life situations, with the oughtness, obligations, and rights in life. Sternberg identified and analyzed four concepts that might serve as a philosophic foundation for nursing ethics. Each of the four is now used, or their meanings exist, in nursing practice. They are different philosophically and have disparate connotations and implications. The four concepts are *code*, the present instrument utilized by the profession to promulgate ethical standards; *contract* (not defined by Sternberg); *context*, where the arena in which ethical conflict occurs is the determinant of ethical response; and *covenant*, a formalized agreement between persons to do or not to do something specific. Sternberg did not make clear how contract and covenant differ. The presentation of the concepts and discussion of their implications are highly informative. They would be useful to all nurses concerned with defining or delineating nursing ethics. They could also be useful to those who teach ethics in the context of nursing.

Swedish investigators Norberg, Norberg, and Bexell (1980) used both empirical and philosophic inquiry to study ethical problems arising in the feeding of patients with advanced dementia. The condition of patients with advanced dementia may deteriorate to a point where spoon feeding is no longer possible or safe. The alternative of forced feeding by intubation has its own evils and dangers. Starvation is unacceptable. This real and common ethical dilemma for nurses involved in the care of patients with extremely advanced dementia provoked the study.

Norberg, Norberg, and Bexell (1980) made careful observations over a four-week period on wards where long-term geriatric patients were provided care. During these observations, the investigators held repeated discussion with the nurses caring for the patients. The observations and discussions provided material for philosophic analysis. From this analysis, five conflicting demands that created ethical dilemmas for nurses were identified. The consequences of the dilemmas and avenues for resolution were explored. The report of the study was too brief and lacked the detailed discussion of the conflicting demands of dilemmas necessary for a substantive contribution to nursing knowledge. The investigators were concerned with calling attention to the existence of dilemmas and to the need for further study of them. There was insufficient detail and explication in the report. It did, however, provide one model for beginning philosophic inquiry of nursing ethics.

There is a great need for continued systematic inquiry from many approaches to the study of ethics, ethical dilemmas, conflicting demands that defy resolution, and nursing ethics as conceived and lived by nurses. Philosophic inquiry has been used very little in the vital area of nursing ethics. Such inquiry is greatly needed. Philosophic inquiry has been used to a greater extent, and for a longer period of time, in research on nursing education.

PHILOSOPHY OF NURSING EDUCATION

The earliest identified philosophic inquiry done by a nurse was that of Newton (1949). It was an investigation of the philosophy of nursing education of Florence Nightingale. The study was based on interpretation of Nightingale's concepts of reality, man, God, religion, standards, means and ends, goals, education, and nursing education. Nightingale's beliefs were then related by Newton to three schools of philosophical thought—scholasticism, idealism, and pragmatism. The conclusion Newton drew was that Nightingale was eclectic and quite pragmatic. The investigation provided insight into the philosophic tenets basic to Nightingale's activities and prescriptions. The prescriptions have had a lasting impact on American nursing. Newton's contribution has been to identify their philosophic source. Whether the prescriptions are valid for contemporary nursing depends upon the usefulness of pragmatics as a major mode for decisions and whether the pragmatically based prescriptions from the 19th century are still valid.

Nightingale was also a focus for Barritt's (1971/1972) investigation. Barritt analyzed Nightingale's writings to study the values that could be identified regarding nursing education. Barritt used the headings for the National League for Nursing criteria for appraisal of baccalaureate and higher degree programs in nursing as a taxonomy for the study. The Nightingale values and those of contemporary baccalaureate education in nursing were highly correlated, according to Barritt.

History and philosophy overlap when history of ideas or values are at issue. The Barritt study is not primarily concept clarification; it is more a study of premises and oughts. It is a demonstration of continuity over time in nursing. Schuyler's (1975/1976) study of Nightingale and Louise Schuyler used history and philosophy to delineate the philosophies of nursing education of these two nurses. Their philosophies of nursing education were presented in the context of their era and their general philosophies of life. Schuyler the investigator also related the two nurses' views to reigning philosophies of education of their times. Schuyler's inquiry added little to further understanding of Nightingale beyond that provided by Newton (1949) or Barritt (1971/1972). There are other historical figures in American nursing that warrant study besides Louise Schuyler. The study does not have general usefulness for nursing.

Philosophic inquiry of nursing education that coupled such inquiry with empirical study also was found. Both philosophic inquiry and an empirical study were done by Vaillot (1962) on commitment to nursing. From an existential viewpoint, Vaillot sought to resolve the opposition or separation between the Habenstein and Christ (1955) classifications of nurses as traditionalizers and utilizers. Vaillot rejected the either/or classification. She identified commitment as the critical element in nursing. She characterized nursing education as a passage from existence to being. Vaillot's analysis of the Habenstein and Christ concepts of traditionalizer and utilizer was dialectic. Synthesis was accomplished with the concept of commitment. Commitment became the essential good for Vaillot. Vaillot also did an empirical study of the worlds of students in nursing. She asked students in collegiate, diploma, and practical schools of nursing to answer with whom they identified and what their appraisal of nursing as a profession was. For Vaillot, education for commitment to nursing was the essential and ultimate good for nursing education. Commitment was identified as crucial for authentic being as a nurse. The means to this end was not explicated. It is not at all clear why the empirical study was done or how it contributed to the advancement of Vaillot's thesis or to nursing knowledge.

Commitment, along with *caring* and *presence,* were identified by Nelson (1977/1978) in a philosophic inquiry of ideas in nursing literature that corresponded to ideas of the existentialist philosophers Martin Buber and Gabriel Marcel. The intersubjectivity in the nurse-patient encounter was identified. Commitment was viewed as necessary for selfhood in nursing. This view is identical to that of Vaillot. Commitment was also deemed by both Vaillot and Nelson to be vital to the future of the nursing profession.

Caring was viewed as essential to self-actualization of the nurse. Nelson also thought is was essential for rendering care in the interests of the other. Presence, or being there subjectively, was also considered to be essential for care. Presence, however, created a potential for difficulty in that it required self-disclosure and availability. Nelson's discussion raised questions that beg answers through philosophic study. Are there limits to commitment, caring, or presence? How much is it reasonable to expect a nurse, as nurse, to open up to a patient or client? Is there such a thing as a professional relationship? Is it different from other human relationships? If so, what are the differences? What are the implications? What are realistic expectations? What are the norms? What are the limits? Inquiry in this area has not yet been done; it should be done.

CONCEPTS, VALUES, AND PROCESSES

A Greek nurse explained the Greek derivation of the word "philosophy" (Lanara, 1976). The word literally means "love of wisdom." Lanara viewed philosophy as helping one to develop a coherent world view, one that makes sense of everyday experience. This world view was described as an outlook; a body of values; and a synthesis of spiritual, moral, humanitarian, and social values by Lanara.

The heading *Philosophy, Nursing* in the *International Nursing Index* is used for listing articles on nursing theory, personal or institutional philosophies of nursing, concepts, and much else. The increase in the number of listings under the heading is quite striking since the first volume of the index appeared in 1966. The increase attests to more conceptual analyses and to concern for meanings in nursing. Part of the search for meanings is through philosophic analysis of concepts, discovery or extraction of concepts from literature, and search for values.

Six investigations of concepts, values, or meanings that qualify as philosophic research were found. The six investigations are only similar in that they are philosophic inquiries and were done by nurses. The six investigators have begun work that must be done to make manifest a nursing perspective or world view, if one indeed does exist.

The first study in this group is a study of empathy by Zderad (1968). As a philosopher, Zderad inquired into the nature of empathy, its ingredients, and processes. She also delineated the synthesis process by which her construct, empathy, was developed. The description of the synthesis process is a contribution to nursing methodology. It was Zderad's logical contention that nursing requires both the objective view, as found in science, and the subjective view. The subjective view was thought to be essential for knowing in the intersubjectivity of the nurse-patient relationship. Subjectivity, as evident in phenomenology, also was considered valuable because of the very nature of nursing practice. Nursing practice is concerned with both objective and subjective realities of the human beings involved—nurses and patients. Empathy, for Zderad, requires subjectivity. It is lived.

Phenomenology is a philosophy and a method of inquiry. The method is used to describe and understand events or other phenomena as they are experienced and lived. Subjective meanings and intuition are used to understand the experiencing as lived. Phenomenology can be used to elucidate the experience of illness as lived, for example. Nurses must seek to understand human responses to illness, if they are to nurse effectively. Phenomenology may contribute to the understanding. It was Zderad's thesis that empathy cannot be understood or studied solely from objective scientific processes. Empathy may be a learned skill; it is also a philosophic stance expressed through art in nursing. Synthesis of objectivity and subjectivity occurs in the nursing act. There is synthesis of several realities and synthesis of art, science, and experience. Knowledge development for nursing practice must explore methods for synthesis. The Zderad study is a contribution in this area. It is an example of the process of synthesis.

Health and its various meanings were the objects of Smith's (1981) investigation. The study was a critical analysis of the foundations of various meanings of health. Smith sought to explicate, clarify, and extend knowledge by logic and reasoning and presented four different ideas of health that she found in the literature. She tested them by the method of testing ideas in philosophic inquiry, that of critical discussion. The four models of health identified by Smith were:

1. eudaimonistic—health as a general well-being and self-actualization;
2. adaptive—health as a condition of capability for effective interaction with the physical and the social environment,
3. role performance—health as measured by effective role performance; and
4. clinical—health as the absence of morbid physical or mental condition.

Smith argued that nurses need to think of health from the adaptive or eudaimonistic orientation and thereby to become guardians of the quality of life in the community.

Accepting this function for nurses appeals as a laudable ideal, but it would be difficult to realize. Realistically, there is a myriad of variables that affect the condition of existence of any individual or group. It is totally unrealistic to expect nurses to be responsible for, to be able to treat, or to manage all the variables of existence. Although it is impossible to define operationally or to evaluate quality of life, this should not rule out an argument for rejection of the clinical model of health for nursing. Smith's critical discussion of the four models provided nurses with a clearer view of the differences and the range of models of health. It did not explain how the models could be used. Further work is needed to show how the elucidation of the models can lead to further development of nursing knowledge or practice. The Smith study did provide a useful approximation for the beginning of order in the amibiguous meanings of the term "health."

Healing was the focus of Homberg's (1980) inquiry, in which roots of healing were identified in the Bible. Homberg concluded that the biblical tradition of the healing power of respect for human worth and dignity, of interpersonal relationships, of community, and of meal fellowship have parallels in contemporary nursing. The significance of this conclusion is unclear. The observed parallels to biblical tradition are not unique to nursing. It is reasonable to expect some biblical influence on nursing, given the centuries of involvement of religious communities in nursing. The study does indicate some conditions for, or components of, healing. This is useful for nursing.

A value may be a subject for philosophic inquiry. Raya (1975) characterized the nursing profession as a treasury of values. What these values are and how they are manifest has not been delineated or investigated. Only one study, of one nursing value, was found for this review. It is that of an investigation of heroism as a value (Lanara, 1974). (This doctoral dissertation also was published as a book in both Greek and English; see Lanara, 1981.) With the purpose of enriching and redefining nursing philosophy, Lanara (1974) examined the concepts and images of heroism as they related to nursing. Philosophy, including primary sources from classical Greece and the Byzantine period, and philosophic nursing literature was used. In addition, writings of Nightingale and statements on nursing from the International Council of Nursing, the World Health Organization, and nursing leaders were analyzed. The values of responsibility, respect for human dignity, and sacrifice were illustrated in relation to the concept heroism. The concept heroism was deemed relevant to nursing situations. The heroism of love for fellow human beings in need of care was an idea Lanara (1974) found to permeate nursing philosophy. Nursing philosophy was viewed by Lanara (1976) as a reservoir of values that can provide criteria for choices nurses must make for the benefit of the served other and the living spirit of care. Lanara's concept of heroism, which encompasses respect for human dignity, is somewhat different from the common American concept of heroism. The element of sacrific elucidated by Lanara (1974) raises for nurses questions similar to those identified earlier in this review about commitment. Commitment and sacrifice have been expectations in nursing. The extent to which they are current expectations remains to be studied. Meanings, norms, and limits must also be investigated.

Meaning in suffering, treated as a nursing dilemma, was the subject of another investigation. Kreidler (1978/1979) used an existential and spiritual framework to articulate an approach intended to humanize the nurse's encounter with those who suffer. The approach was offered as an alternative to the need for self-control and control of others to protect against feelings of helplessness. In the investigation, the terms *spiritual, existential,* and *suffering* were clarified from contemporary literature in philosophy. Nursing literature on spirituality and existential themes also was examined. A conceptualization of human beings as spiritual persons needing to find meaning in life and in suffering was explicated. Transcendence was considered a desirable potential that might be realized, depending upon how one viewed and used suffering. A nurse's personal philosophy was thought by Kreidler (1978/1979) to be important for facing the suffering of others. It was also thought to be important for its consequences in nurse-patient interactions. The Kreidler study should be valuable for nurses involved in care of patients with cancer or other long term or catastrophic health problems. It may also be of more general use for understanding nursing. It could help nurses recognize or formulate their personal philosophies. It could help in understanding or patterning behavior.

The sixth study in the group was a study of a process, in contrast to a construct or value. The subject of the study was judgment. Doona (1975) sought to clarify the judgment process in nursing. She contributed a theory of judgment to systematized nursing knowledge (Doona, 1976). Doona (1975) reviewed and critically analyzed the implied or stated views of judgment of major philosophers. She identified two pivotal thinkers, Saint Thomas Aquinas and John Dewey. The theories of judgment of these philosophers were synthesized by Doona to form a new theory. Phases of judgment and varieties of judgment such as common sense, speculative, and pragmatic, were considered in the context of nursing. Doona's (1975) theory of judgment was delineated in a paradigm and operationally defined. The study's consequences for improvement in decision making in nursing practice could be considerable. Doona (1976) demonstrates the practical utility that may accrue from philosophic inquiry.

METHODOLOGY AND NURSING

Methodology is a branch of logic dealing with principles of procedure. Principles of procedure specify how knowledge is produced and the criteria for its acceptance as knowledge. Methodology is the study, description, explanation, and justification of methods. Five philosophic studies by nurses were found. They can be grouped by their common focus on methodology and nursing. In other respects they are quite dissimilar. They are reviewed in chronological order.

The first study, by Paterson (1971), proposed a method for nursing research developed from synthesis, application, and conceptualization of philosophic ideas in relation to Paterson's beliefs about what she terms "professional clinical nursing." Paterson identified her study as methodological inquiry directed at understanding the process, rather than the products, of scientific inquiry. "Nursology" was Paterson's term to designate the study of nursing aimed at the development of nursing theory. Paterson's method of nursology was presented in a five-phase model. The model was a description of a subjective-objective method of study Paterson thought was essential for, and specific to, the humanistic nature of nursing. Concern for the humanistic traditions of nursing is pervasive in nursing literature. Many nurses think the emphasis on science and on the generality and objectivity that characterize science threaten nursing practice traditions. For some, scientific objectivity vitiates or violates the humanitarian essence of nursing. Polarization of science and humanitarianism seems to be occurring. Philosophers strive to provide the synoptic view. Paterson's inquiry is an example of the synthesis that must be achieved in the development of nursing knowledge. If such knowledge is to serve as the base for practice, science and humanitarianism must be synthesized. Paterson's inquiry offers one model for the process of synthesis. There must be continued study of the process of synthesis. There is need for a synoptic view of what are treated as disparate areas of knowing in nursing. As manifest in nursing practice, these disparate areas must create a whole.

Another study to clarify the process for theory development in nursing was that of Walker (1971a). In Walker's inquiry and in an article based upon it (Walker, 1971b), nursing was considered in the context of discipline. Discipline, defined as a community of scholars who share a common orientation to a domain of inquiry, and to the principles for the production of knowledge, is not generally understood in nursing. The Walker (1971a) inquiry in the context of discipline demonstrated the difference between knowledge-development procedures and principles and the nature of nursing as a practice. Nursing practice has as goals the health and welfare of human beings. Nursing, as practiced, is a humanistic resource for health. Knowledge-development procedures serve as means for extending knowledge. They are independent of the uses of knowledge or a practice.

Whether nursing is or should become a discipline remains to be explored. There is some evidence of communality in thinking in nursing as noted by Donaldson and Crowely (1978). However, as Donaldson and Crowley point out, there is no single method of inquiry in nursing. Science, history, and philosophy are methods of inquiry that seem essential in nursing. What is the structure for a body of knowledge that is produced by such distinctive approaches? What synthetic processes are required to create a meaningful whole? The substantive and methodological structures for a nursing discipline need to be explicated and the work of Donaldson and Crowley (1978) and of Walker (1971a) and Carper (1975/1976) continued.

Traditional science as a threat to nursing values was evident in the Taddy (1975/1976) investigation. Taddy noted that examination of the historical development, the assumptions, the concepts, the prejudices, and the methods of traditional science imperil the preservation of the unique and personal character of human beings. Taddy found evidence in nursing literature of resistence to the potential loss, through generalization, of the human aspects of persons. She felt that nurses, as scientists, must reconcile objectivity and generality with being humane, with subjectivity, and with individualism. Knowledge about humans generated from objective and subjective studies is essential knowledge for effective nursing practice. What Taddy identified as at issue is: What views of humans are appropriate, for what purpose, and for what questions? These are questions nurse investigators must consider and investigate as philosophers. The pervading traditions of nursing would seem to require preservation of all that the concept person has connoted in nursing. Exactly what it does connote or what it is intended to connote remain unstudied areas for which philosophic inquiry is a useful method of investigation. Other methods of inquiry should be examined to ascertain their usefulness and compatibility with nursing views of human beings.

A brief treatise on nursing and methodology was found in a letter to the editor of *Nursing Research*. The contribution of the author (Zbilut, 1978) warrants mention in this review. Zbilut noted that there were epistemologic constraints to the development of a theory of nursing. Zbilut claimed that viable models depended upon social decision for validation, that it is not possible to create viable models or to assume perspectives incongruent with envisioned practice. Models of envisioned practice must submit to the test of social decision for viability. Zbilut identified four "habits of thinking" (p. 128) in viewing human nature. These are:

1. empiriological—experiential (scientific research and personal experience),
2. empirical—metaphenomenal (hypothesis, theory, law),
3. philosophical—metaphenomenal (human contingencies of man's existence viewed with regard to a space-time axis), and
4. philosophical-transcendental (formalities which embrace being with precision from the space-time axis).

According to Zbilut, participation is the only way some things can be known. Knowing another person as a fellow human being, for example, cannot be achieved from objectivity and mere observation. Zbilut's position endorses phenomenology and indicates limits of the empirical-metaphenomenal habit of thinking for producing a theory of nursing. It is useful to have Zbilut's brief identification of the four habits of thinking. All four have been used to seek nursing knowledge. The four habits encompass

the approaches advocated by Donaldson and Crowley (1978). The taxonomy accommodates Paterson's (1971) nursology. What remains to be
developed is a methodology of nursing for the integration of the various
views of human nature resulting from the different habits of thinking. There
is also need to ponder the habit of thinking that can produce the socially
congruent viable model of nursing.

The investigations and considerations of methodology have raised
questions about the particular nature of nursing practice. They have raised
questions about the knowledge base essential and sufficient for that practice. How nurses think, their values as a collective, their reflections, and
what counts as good must be studied further through philosophic inquiry
and discourse. At present, a case has been made for scientific, philosophic,
and historical research in nursing. Emphasis has been on scientific research. The usefulness of the generalizations that are the products of
science seems not to be questioned. What has been overlooked, except by
philosophers in nursing, is the continuing need for knowing the particular
that is required by the nature of the human responsibilities entailed in
effective nursing care. What is also to be sought is the wholeness in
knowing. A search for nursing meanings, begun with Zderad's (1968)
study of empathy, Lanara's (1974) study of heroism, and Kreidler's (1978/
1979) study of suffering must be continued and expanded. There is also a
need to confront complex, comprehensive questions. There is need to
examine, for example, what it means to be compassionate, humane, and
caring toward patients. There is need to explicate the nursing meaning of
person, or the meaning of "being there," or the meaning of dignity.
Philosophic inquiry is required for these tasks.

SUMMARY

Criteria for the evaluation of philosophic inquiry in nursing are logic,
clarity, and the significance of the questions or problems for nursing. An
additional criterion might be the meaningfulness of the inquiry for enlight-
enment and for ordering understandings and meanings in nursing. On all of
these criteria, the relatively few philosophic inquiries by nurses are generally acceptable and make a contribution to nursing research. They begin to
explicate and clarify meanings from existing knowledge. There are very
few nurses who have become philosophers. It is essential that this pool be

enlarged. Continuing inquiry is needed to examine and explicate other meanings, to further methodology for nursing knowledge, and to identify and explicate nursing values and ethics. The domain of human experience in illness must be explored further to provide knowledge vital for nursing practice. Practice requires a synthesis of the various ways of knowing. This synthesis must be manifest in the ways of being, in doing for and with another person.

Too many of the studies reviewed here were doctoral dissertations that did not result in publication. The reasons for this are not known. Perhaps it is part of a more general picture of the fate of a proportion of dissertations. It could be, however, that review panels and editors of journals are not familiar with philosophic inquiry or that the purposes for which a journal exists are too narrow to accommodate reports of philosophic inquiry. It was abundantly clear to the reviewer that indexing systems in nursing are not very useful for cataloguing the comprehensive scope of philosophic inquiries. The indexing systems reflect the absence of a comprehensive, coherent taxonomy for nursing research. The problem is a general one for nursing research. It is particularly acute for research that is philosophic.

Finally, it is easy to differentiate science, history, and philosophy in the abstract. Ultimately, in the human experience of knowing, they must become a whole. By and large, philosophy has been neglected by nurses, or it has been considered only superficially. The neglect and superficiality are a detriment to nursing and nursing-knowledge development. The potential of philosophic inquiry for nursing is largely unrealized.

REFERENCES

Applegate, M. I. Moral decisions in selected clinical nursing practice situations (Doctoral dissertation, Columbia University Teachers College, 1981). *Dissertation Abstracts International,* 1981, *42,* 1818B. (University Microfilms No. 81–22, 930)

Barritt, E. R. B. Florence Nightingale's values regarding nursing education (Doctoral dissertation, Ohio State University, 1971). *Dissertation Abstracts International,* 1972, *32,* 4029B. (University Microfilms No. 72–4418)

Beckstrand, J. The notion of a practice theory and the relationship of scientific and ethical knowledge to practice. *Research in Nursing and Health,* 1978, *1,* 131–136.

Beckstrand, J. A critique of several conceptions of practice theory. *Research in Nursing and Health,* 1980, *3,* 69–79.

Carper, B. Fundamental patterns of knowing in nursing (Doctoral dissertation, Columbia University Teachers College, 1975). *Dissertation Abstracts International*, 1976, *36*, 4941B. (University Microfilms No. 76–7772)

Carper, B. Fundamental patterns of knowing in nursing. *Advances in Nursing Science*, 1978, *1*(1), 13–23.

Curtin, L. L. The nurse as advocate: A philosophical foundation for nursing. *Advances in Nursing Science*, 1979, *1*(3), 1–10.

Davis, A. Ethical dilemmas in nursing: A survey. *Western Journal of Nursing Research*, 1981, *3*, 397–400.

Donaldson, S. K., & Crowley, D. M. The discipline of nursing. *Nursing Outlook*, 1978, *26*, 113–120.

Doona, M. E. A philosophical study of judgment for use in nursing (Doctoral dissertation, Boston University, 1975). *Dissertation Abstracts International*, 1975, *36*, 1369A. (University Microfilms No. 75–20, 918)

Doona, M. E. The judgment process in nursing. *Image*, 1976, *8*, 27–29.

Flew, A. Preface. In J. Speake (Ed.), *A dictionary of philosophy*. New York: St. Martin's, 1979.

Habenstein, R. N., & Christ, E. A. *Professionalizer, traditionalizer and utilizer*. Columbia: University of Missouri Press, 1955.

Homberg, M. A. Biblical roots of healing (Doctoral dissertation, Columbia University Teachers College, 1980). *Dissertation Abstracts International*, 1980, *41*, 1310B. (University Microfilms No. 80–22, 117)

Ketefian, S. Critical thinking, educational preparation and development of moral judgment among selected groups of practicing nurses. *Nursing Research*, 1981, *30*, 98–103. (a)

Ketefian, S. Moral reasoning and moral behavior among selected groups of practicing nurses. *Nursing Research*, 1981, *30*, 171–176. (b)

Kneller, G. F. *Science as a human endeavor*. New York: Columbia University Press, 1978.

Kreidler, M. C. Meaning in suffering: A nursing dilemma (Doctoral dissertation, Columbia University Teachers College, 1978). *Dissertation Abstracts International*, 1979, *39*, 4813B. (University Microfilms No. 79–09001)

Lanara, V. A. Heroism as a nursing value (Doctoral dissertation, Columbia University, 1974). *Dissertation Abstracts International*, 1974, *35*, 2848B. (University Microfilms No. 74–26, 597)

Lanara, V. A. Philosophy of nursing and current nursing problems. *International Nursing Review*, 1976, *23*, 48–54.

Lanara, V. A. *Heroism as a missing value*. Athens, Greece: Publications Sisterhood Eviniki, 1981.

Mooney, M. M. The ethical component of nursing theory: An analysis of ethical components in four nursing theories. *Image*, 1980, *12*, 7–9.

Murphy, C. P. Levels of moral reasoning in a selected group of nursing practitioners (Doctoral dissertation, Columbia University Teachers College, 1976). *Dissertation Abstracts International*, 1977, *38*, 593B. (University Microfilms No. 77–16, 684)

Nelson, Sr. M. J. The thoughts of Martin Buber and Gabriel Marcel: Implications for existential encounters in nursing (Doctoral dissertation, Columbia University Teachers College, 1977). *Dissertation Abstracts International*, 1978, *39*, 222B. (University Microfilms No. 78–21, 826)

Newton, M. E. *Florence Nightingale's philosophy of life and education*. Unpublished doctoral dissertation, Stanford University, 1949.

Norberg, A., Norberg, B., & Bexell, G. Ethical problems in feeding patients with advanced dementia. *British Medical Journal*, 1980, *281*, 847–848.

Paterson, J. S. From a philosophy of clinical nursing to a method of nursology. *Nursing Research*, 1971, *20*, 143–146.

Phenix, P. H. *Realms of meaning*. New York: McGraw-Hill, 1964.

Raya, A. C. Psychiatric nursing: A conceptual approach. A textbook for Greece (Doctoral dissertation, Columbia University, 1975). *Dissertation Abstracts International*, 1975, *36*, 1149B-1150B. (University Microfilms No. 75–20, 233)

Rorty, R. *Philosophy and the mirror of nature*. Princeton: Princeton University Press, 1979.

Schuyler, C. B. Molders of modern nursing: Florence Nightingale and Louise Shuyler (Doctoral dissertation, Columbia University Teachers College, 1975) *Dissertation Abstracts International*, 1976, *37*, 1179B. (University Microfilms No. 76–20, 875)

Silva, M. C. Philosophy, science, theory: Interrelationships and implications for nursing research. *Image*, 1977, *9*, 59–63.

Smith, J. A. The idea of health: A philosophical inquiry. *Advances in Nursing Science*, 1981, *3*(3), 43–50.

Sternberg, M. J. The search for a conceptual framework as a philosophical basis for nursing ethics: An examination of code, contract, context and covenant. *Military Medicine*, 1979, *144*, 9–22.

Taddy, Sr. J. A philosophical inquiry into existential philosophy as an approach for nursing (Doctoral dissertation, University of Pittsburgh, 1975). *Dissertation Abstracts International*, 1976, *36*, 1369B. (University Microfilms No. 76–14, 173)

Vaillot, Sr. M. C. *Commitment to nursing: A philosophic investigation*. Phildelphia: Lippincott, 1962.

Walker, L. O. Nursing as a discipline (Doctoral dissertation, Indiana University, 1971). *Dissertation Abstracts International*, 1971, *32*, 3459B. (University Microfilms No. 72–1528) (a)

Walker, L. O. Toward a clearer understanding of the concept of nursing theory. *Nursing Research*, 1971, *20*, 428–435. (b)

Zbilut, J. P. Epistemologic constraints to the development of a theory of nursing. *Nursing Research*, 1978, *27*, 128–129.

Zderad, L. T. A concept of empathy (Doctoral dissertation, Georgetown University, 1968). *Dissertation Abstracts International*, 1968, *29*, 936A-937A. (University Microfilms No. 68–12, 814)

Index

Index